OXFORD MEDICAL PUBLICATIONS

Spinal Cord Dysfunction
Volume II
Intervention and Treatment

Spinal Cord Dysfunction

Volume II
Intervention and Treatment

Edited by

L. S. Illis

Consultant Neurologist, Wessex Neurological Centre,
Southampton General Hospital
Clinical Senior Lecturer in Neurology,
University of Southampton Medical School

Oxford   New York   Tokyo
OXFORD UNIVERSITY PRESS
1992

Oxford University Press, Walton Street, Oxford OX2 6DP

Oxford New York Toronto
Delhi Bombay Calcutta Madras Karachi
Petaling Jaya Singapore Hong Kong Tokyo
Nairobi Dar es Salaam Cape Town
Melbourne Auckland
and associated companies in
Berlin Ibadan

Oxford is a trade mark of Oxford University Press

Published in the United States
by Oxford University Press, New York

A catalogue record for this book is available from the British Library

Library of Congress Cataloging in Publication Data
(Revised for vol. II)
Spinal cord dysfunction.
(Oxford medical publications)
Includes bibliographies and index.
Contents: [1] Assessment—Intervention and treatment
1. Spinal cord—Wounds and injuries.
I. Illis, L. S. (Leon S.)
RD594.3.S665   1988   617'.482075   87-31490
ISBN 0-19-261624-2 (v. I)
ISBN 0-19-261787-7 (v. II)

Typeset by Joshua Associates Ltd, Oxford
Printed in Great Britain by
Courier International Ltd, East Kilbride

Foreword

Sir George Bedbrook

Here is a communication on spinal cord injuries which, like Volume I of the series, is new and important. This second volume of a proposed three volume series on the spinal cord and its response to dysfunction is a credit to its distinguished contributors and, particularly, to its editor, whose work I have known of for some years.

Having had the opportunity of reading that material presented in the manuscript, it is undoubtedly a volume to be read and re-read by all medical scientists involved in the intervention of spinal cord dysfunction. The old criticism of therapeutic nihilism, so common in earlier decades, should now be discarded permanently as the advances of the last decades are vigorously applied.

As the editor indicates in his Preface, this volume contains only some of the aspects of functional pathology as it affects spinal man. With the gradual build up of experimental models, the recently improved pathological knowledge from neuropathological laboratories, and the functional neurological information thus available, there is no doubt that the concept of clinical manipulation affecting the outcome, as outlined in this volume, is not only therapeutically possible, but has already become, in part, practically possible.

Spinal cord neurology for patients changes with time and conditions, as those small number of clinicians heavily involved over the last four decades know only too well. Thus, the theoretical and applied science now reported helps to prove the plasticity of the human nervous system. This book will be enjoyed by those who seek to improve practical care, for the contributors have discussed the various arguments and scientific data extremely well. It is a pity, however, that the arguments concerning initial care as it affects surgical thought have not by now, half a century after comprehensive units were established, been more scientifically settled, simply because on both sides of the debate, with very few exceptions, the pathological knowledge now available has not been used and the use of large multi-centre trials with independent assessment has not been undertaken. Dr W. El Masri's attempt at assessment appears fair and equitable as knowledge stands at the present time.

At this time some hundred or more comprehensive services are active in which the fundamentals of secondary prevention, so well practised since the advent of Units in the United Kingdom, United States, and Canada by famous pioneers such as Munro, Botterel, and Guttmann, are now well established by scientific proof. Re-assessment of such fundamentals is helped by the scientific knowledge amassed in this volume. For example, Wise Young's chapter on therapy, where corticosteroids and calcium blockers can be practically applied, since the knowledge of intra-cellular and extra-cellular exchanges after injury has been well documented for clinical application.

Preventive medicine has long since entered the field of early and late care with the knowledge now displayed and revealed. Dr Illis has given foundation to practical, vigorous management, and thus he and his co-workers have materially helped in the endless struggle to rehabilitate spinal man.

As the future evolves, advances in cellular chemistry will certainly help primary prevention, if only to a small, but significant, degree. That is one of the final frontiers as it was in so many other medical states now vanished—a frontier that needs not only scientific work by medical scientists but by other community disciplines where as yet prevention plays but a small part in the reduction of disability. Spinal cord injury primary prevention is a multi-factorial matter needing the co-operative multi-disciplinary activity of engineers of various professions, of political analysts, of legislators, and early application by professional educators as well as an increasing interest by those medical scientists involved in the early care of spinal cord injuries. No longer is primary prevention the field of health scientists or immunologists. Already some centres have shown that primary prevention is a practicality in up to 30 per cent of present figures, by passive and educative measures as well as better care between the site of accident and admission to a formal spinal injury comprehensive service.

In the Foreword to Volume I of this series, Dr Patrick Wall raised the question as to whether rehabilitation really did apply neuroscience in its endeavours to help patients. This volume certainly espouses or encourages the concept and thus supports a real hope for the future: complete restoration of those afflicted by spinal cord and perhaps cauda equina injury.

In all, therefore, this volume makes a real contribution in a number of fields related to spinal cord dysfunction. Furthermore each chapter has adequate references for the serious student of spinal cord injury. Undoubtedly this volume marks a major milestone in the application of our knowledge of spinal man and goes far in dispersing that pessimism still common in some of the medical disciplines involved. Let me re-emphasize that this is a volume, as was the first, quite different to those text books which have already been published in the area of spinal cord dysfunction.

Preface

The purpose of this book is to bring together experts in various fields of treatment and management of abnormal function following a lesion or disease of the spinal cord. The relatively small size of the volume in no way reflects the enormous problem of spinal dysfunction. In the United States of America over ten thousand victims per year of spinal cord injury will incur costs of 1.7 billion (1974) dollars over their lifetime. Another example of the size of the problem can be seen by the fact that in Britain alone there are 250 000 wheelchair users, of whom 13 000 are spinal injured persons, 60 000 are patients with multiple sclerosis, and 15 000 are patients with spina bifida. If the size of this book does not reflect the size of the problem, it reflects the present situation with regard to treatment of spinal cord dysfunction. Hopefully, this rather pessimistic attitude will change in the future.

Spinal cord dysfunction refers to abnormal function of the spinal cord as a result of injury or disease. The most extreme example of breakdown of function is seen in spinal injury in Man where a lesion, often limited in both space and in time, produces a disastrous and apparently incurable effect. In a disease process, the disturbed function produced by a lesion or multiple lesions is complicated by the ongoing process of the disease, whereas in an apparently static disturbance such as spinal cord injury the features of spinal cord dysfunction are more easily analysed. However, a second 'hidden' lesion may have been sustained. Even in disease processes, each little lesion may produce, in effect, a deafferentation of part of the central nervous system. Many of the effects following both disease and injury are the same, and may respond to similar therapy, although some of the problems are relevant only to trauma. Discussing these together may, hopefully, be of benefit to practising neurologists, clinical neurophysiologists, specialists in rehabilitation, and research workers.

The emphasis here is on intervention. However, identifiable gaps in the volume include, for example, the treatment of pressure sores, which really lies outside the scope of this work. The reason for these gaps is that the intention of the book is not so much to present a factual story of treatment as to suggest a concept. The concept is that the damage produced by a spinal lesion is, theoretically, amenable to clinical manipulation which will effect *outcome*. Eventually, current research into regeneration and transplantation in the central nervous system will bear fruit in terms of treatment of patients; but even this will not preclude the types of treatment discussed in this volume. It is hoped that the reviews presented here will suggest further research directed to the understanding and treatment of spinal dysfunction, and will stimulate interest in the relatively neglected field of restorative or functional neurology.

There have been more studies, both experimental and on patients, in the last ten years than in the preceding half century. This is, of course, partly a reflection of the changing views of experimental and applied science, but it is also because of the realization that the so-called 'fixed' deficits of conventional neurology are not immutable (see Vol. I of this series: *Spinal cord dysfunction: assessment*). As a direct result of this gradually changing idea about the nervous system and its reaction to injury, the first quantitative studies are being carried out in therapy in Man.

The first volume on spinal dysfunction discussed assessment. This volume inquires into some specific aspects of spinal dysfunction. The criteria for inclusion were simply those of importance for the patient, such as in the section of specific problems, or those of controversy, such as the problems of early decompression and of early treatment. As in the previous volume, the authors have indicated the difficulties of the possibility of intervention and treatment. Some of the present authors contributed to the first volume, and emphasize, thereby, the earlier theme: that assessment, treatment, and rehabilitation are inseparable.

Finally, the fact that the discussion of intervention and treatment is so brief will, I hope, be seen as a sign of critical appraisal rather than of therapeutic nihilism.

Southampton   L.S.I.
June 1990

Acknowledgement

Firstly, I must acknowledge the authors who have written the chapters in this book and who have taken such trouble to prepare up-to-date reviews. I must also acknowledge the unstinting work of my secretary, Mrs Sally Allan, who has retyped innumerable drafts.

Finally I wish to acknowledge the help given by Peter Banyard of the International Spinal Research Trust and, in particular, his cheerful encouragement that hope (and hard work) will triumph over experience.

The proceeds of the sale of this book are donated, in their entirety, to the International Spinal Research Trust.

Contents

III Behavioural therapy

Contributors

J. Benfield, Duke of Cornwall Spinal Treatment Centre, Odstock Hospital, Salisbury, UK

Aleksandar Berić, Division of Restorative Neurology and Human Neurobiology, Baylor College of Medicine, Houston, USA

J. D. Cole, Department of Clinical Neurophysiology, Wessex Neurological Centre, Southampton General Hospital, Southampton, UK

W. S. El Masri, The Midland Centre for Spinal Injuries, Institute of Orthopaedics, Oswestry, UK

G. J. Fellows, National Spinal Injuries Centre, Stoke Mandeville Hospital, UK

H. L. Frankel, National Spinal Injuries Centre, Stoke Mandeville Hospital, UK

B. P. Gardner, National Spinal Injuries Centre, Stoke Mandeville Hospital, UK

Robert R. Hansebout, St Joseph's Hospital Spinal Centre and McMaster University, Hamilton, Ontario, Canada

L. S. Illis, Wessex Neurological Centre, Southampton General Hospital, and University of Southampton Medical School, Southampton, UK

C. J. Mathias, Department of Medicine, St Mary's Hospital and Medical School/Imperial College, and University Department of Clinical Neurology, Institute of Neurology, Queen Square, London, UK

D. V. Meerkotter, Institute of Orthopaedics, Oswestry, UK

Theo Mulder, Department of Research and Development, St Maartenskliniek, Nijmegen, The Netherlands

P. Rainsbury, Bourn Hall Clinic, Bourn, Cambridge, UK

E. M. Sedgwick, Department of Clinical Neurophysiology, Wessex Neurological Centre, Southampton General Hospital, and University of Southampton Medical School, Southampton, UK

Wise Young, Department of Neurosurgery, New York University Medical Centre, New York, USA

Introduction

L. S. Illis

The main research drive towards a cure for spinal injury will undoubtedly have an effect on the understanding and potential for treatment of all types of spinal dysfunction. Unfortunately, at present there is no evidence for regeneration of axons in the central nervous system of adult mammals. Growth inhibition, whether because of the innate characteristics of adult nerve cells or because of powerful inhibitory factors expressed by glia, is a major field of regeneration research. If such regeneration does become a possibility then further problems will become apparent, including those of target recognition. A second approach, which is not mutually exclusive with the first, depends on the recognition that neurological deficit is not entirely a direct lesion-induced event but is a reflection of the reaction of the nervous system to the lesion. The reaction includes sprouting, unmasking, alteration of excitation and inhibition, and chemical changes, particularly of neuro-modulation. This was dealt with in the previous volume *Spinal cord dysfunction: assessment* and is the basis of restorative neurology; the recognition of dynamic changes in the development of the so-called 'fixed' neurological deficit and manipulation by neurochemical and stimulation methods in order to restore normal functioning.

A third approach is suggested by the early events found in animal models of spinal cord damage. These studies indicated evidence of progressive tissue damage. Metabolic disturbances, the release or activation of toxic substances, ionic shifts, and a fall in blood-flow in the white matter produces and is consistent with continuing damage at the lesion site. Calcium entry into cells interrupts mitochondrial transport and initiates lipid peroxidation, which in turn releases free radicals causing a continuing injury response, resulting in progressive membrane damage, oedema, and a further fall in blood-flow.

Dr Wise Young raises the perplexing question of why these most critical cells possess such apparent auto-destructive tendencies, and reviews the rationale of treating acute spinal cord injury in the context of this question. He suggests that the response of the spinal cord to trauma is part of the general calcium-activated mechanism by which central nervous tissues protect themselves against excessive calcium entry, and discusses the therapeutic implications of this view.

Within a few hours of severe cord trauma, irreversible changes may occur. This is such an important time in the evolution of spinal injury, and the consequences of delay are so severe, that this is dealt with by both Dr Wise Young and Dr Hansebout, with an intentional overlap. Dr Hansebout reviews some of the more recent methods of treatment that are aimed at preventing the progression of changes which occur in the early stages, and describes the alteration in cord blood-flow which may lie at the basis of the rapid, and potentially reversible, deterioration. Local cooling may save tissue, prevent the development of a complete cord section, and influence outcome.

Can the injury response be altered by drug therapy? As I write the National Institute of Neurological Disorders and Stroke (USA) have issued a 'Clinical Alert'. The notice is of the effect of high doses of methylprednisolone, which has been shown to be beneficial in reducing the effects of spinal cord injury if given within eight hours of trauma. The study was a multi-centre (ten centres) study of a randomized, placebo-controlled, double-blind trial, with 162 patients treated with methylprednisolone, 154 patients treated with naloxone, and 171 patients treated with placebo. Naloxone showed no beneficial effect. Significant improvements in both motor and sensory function were seen in patients treated with high-dose methylprednisolone (bolus dose followed by a maintenance dose) compared with those patients who received placebo. The improvement was seen at six weeks and at six months after injury. These improvements were seen only in those patients who had high-dose methylprednisolone treatment within eight hours of the injury. Improvement in function was seen in both complete and incomplete motor and sensory loss. The study showed, in addition, that there was no indication for treating patients with naloxone or with methylprednisolone started more than eight hours after injury. However, the natural history of spinal cord injury still needs to be worked out accurately, starting within hours of the trauma.

Despite years of experience, the problems of surgical intervention continue, with staunch proponents and opponents equally adamant about the efficacy of outcome. Because of the initial progressive nature of spinal cord injury, with the development of haemorrhage, central necrosis, and oedema, many surgeons favour early surgical decompression and stabilization of the vertebral column. Where there is evidence of compression by bone fragments or intervertebral disc, or a severe dislocation (see *Spinal cord dysfunction: assessment*), surgery may produce marked improvement. However, where trauma has produced an apparent complete transection the issue is less clear. This thorny subject is dealt with in detail by Mr El Masri.

The study of the chronic neurological patient has always been of great interest to clinical neurologists and, more recently, to clinical neurophysiologists. The challenges posed are more difficult and more directly related to the organization and breakdown of neurological function than the questions raised in acute diagnostic neurology. The *care* of the chronic neurological patient has not unfortunately attracted the same attention, and although neurologists are slowly coming to accept long-term care as their responsibility, this will never be regarded as mainstream neurology unless research is intimately linked to management and functional neurology, or restorative neurology is identified as such, and not seen merely as the management of complications.

Spasticity, autonomic dysfunction, bladder management, and pain are areas of distress for the patient and extremely fruitful areas for neurological investigation. The problems and potential for therapy are similar regardless of the spinal lesion which has produced the disorder. Fertility, however, is not usually discussed in detail in a work devoted to spinal disorder, although spinal dysfunction frequently includes sexual dysfunction. Unfortunately, the fact that disabled people need sexual relationships just as much as everybody else is frequently overlooked by neurologists. The need for love and sexual intimacy should be discussed freely and should not be regarded as an optional extra; nor should sexual counselling await the patient's request. Many patients are too embarrassed to raise the subject. Until recently most men with complete spinal lesions have been unable to father children because of inability to have intercourse or to ejaculate. Not surprisingly, the failure to achieve children adds considerably to the psychological problems associated with spinal injury and disease. Recently a number of techniques have been developed which overcome the problems of intercourse and ejaculation and the problems of infertility. Disturbances of fertility can be readily understood in terms of damage to functionally specific pathways. However, spasticity, pain, and autonomic dysfunction are not so readily explained on the basis of morphologically distinct pathways, and may be more readily understood in terms of alteration of structure and activity in the undamaged nervous system.

Although many authorities have stated that pain in spinal injury is uncommon, there is no doubt that dysaesthesiae and pain are problems which may be particularly severe in patients with some residual function. Dr Berić estimates that one third of patients complain of pain. Rose *et al*. (1988) reported 69 per cent of a sample of 885 patients with spinal injury who reported pain at or below the level of the lesion at some time since the injury. The site of pain was of a root distribution in 110 patients, in the lower limbs alone in 165 subjects, in the trunk alone in 92, the buttocks alone in 22, and in the abdomen and pelvis alone in 16. In 43 per cent of the sample the pain was constant. The effect of injury on employment is substantial. However, 98 subjects said that it was the severity of their pain and not the paralysis which actually stopped them working, and of those in work 83 per cent said that pain interfered with their work. There was no evidence of resolution of the chronic pain simply with time.

Autonomic disturbance is an important factor in spinal dysfunction, where a large proportion of autonomic outflow may be disrupted and thus produce dissociation from higher regulation. Alteration in cardio-vascular control may affect not only the extent of the initial injury but also reflect the final outcome. Dr Mathias, Dr Frankel, and Dr Cole concentrate on the management of cardio-vascular abnormalities resulting from such dysfunction. Mr Fellows deals with the management of bladder problems. Poor genito-urinary treatment in the early phases may result in disastrous results, whereas careful and logical management should produce improved quality of life and increased life expectancy.

Without careful rehabilitation, which should start with the onset of the lesion, future therapy will be rendered useless and the assessment of such therapy made unnecessarily difficult.

Behavioural therapy warrants a volume, if not an encyclopaedia, of its own. Unfortunately it is impossible to explore all aspects of behavioural therapy, and it would probably not be relevant in any case. Dr Mulder discusses some recent ideas in motor control and learning. In previous chapters the emphasis has been on neurophysiological mechanisms, but here the focus is on human behaviour, and the human organism is seen as a complex self-regulating system which is capable of receiving, processing, and transmitting information and is indissolubly linked with the environment. If rehabilitation is seen as the acquisition and re-acquisition of skills, then the theory of skill acquisition as seen in cognitive experimental psychology is a relevant field of study for therapists.

Dr Mulder deals with the rehabilitation of motor disorders in general rather than concentrating solely on spinal cord dysfunction. There are no clear answers, no array of facts which are immediately applicable in therapeutic situations—rather a theoretical new look at many old problems.

Reference

Rose, M., Robinson, J. E., Ells, P., and Cole, J. D. (1988). Pain following spinal cord injury: results from a postal survey. *Pain*, **34**, 101–2.

I

The acute phase

1

Early decompression of the spinal cord following injury: arguments for and against

W. S. El Masri and D. V. Meerkotter

Introduction

The management of the traumatized spinal cord has remained controversial over the past half century. Arguments for and against each treatment modality exist. Each is equally likely to be adopted or disparaged until possibly all factors hindering spinal cord recovery are identified. Direct comparison between surgery and conservative management in a series of unselected patients would contribute to solving the controversy (Lewis and McKibbin 1974).

The difficulties with design of studies and statistical evaluation of the results should not be underestimated. Problems of designing such comparative clinical studies are to be expected, since, even in the controlled animal studies, reproducibility is not always possible.

The idea that the words of Guttmann should be reiterated almost a decade after his death brings home the stark reality that we have come but a little way in determining the truth in the ever-present conflict over the operative as against the dynamic conservative management of these patients.

The current management varies from a conservative to a surgical approach. Surgery consists of either decompression or stabilization or a combination of both.

Basis of management

Most clinicians base their arguments on clinical experience and belief, as well as on the experimental and clinical work available in the literature. Frankel *et al.* (1969), Bedbrook (1969), Guttmann (1976), Burke *et al.* (1976), and other proponents of conservative management have concluded, following decades of experience, that most of the damage to the spinal cord occurs at the time of the accident, and that surgical decompression is in the majority of cases unlikely to alter the course of events favourably. Spinal cord decompression may result in neurological deterioration which is either transient (Bohlman and Eismont 1981; Gertzbein *et al.* 1988) or permanent

(Morgan *et al.* 1971; Wiberg and Hauge 1988). El Masri *et al.* (in press) believe that this neurological deterioration is probably related to a 'physiological instability' in an injured spinal cord. This 'instability' is possibly due to a combination of spinal cord microvascular alterations, loss of autoregulation, and biochemical and enzymatic changes in patients with impaired autonomic functions.

Furthermore, this instability is not always associated with or directly related to the biomechanical instability of the bony column nor to the decompressive surgery.

It is possible that with extra attention to the haemodynamics of the traumatized patient, neurological deterioration may be reduced or avoided.

The concept of the secondary insult following injury dates back to the early 1950s, when Freeman and Wright (1953) proposed that loss of vascular perfusion secondary to bony encasement of an oedematous haemorrhagic contused spinal cord may cause a secondary injury. Many pharmaceutical agents and surgical procedures were tried in the hope of manipulating favourably this secondary insult.

The drug studies, however, failed to give uniform results: almost all agents have in some study failed to show an effect as tested in one or more laboratories (Collins 1983). Corticosteroids, the commonest clinically used drugs, were demonstrated to improve neurological recovery in animals. Ducker and Hamit (1969), Young and Dexter (1978), and many others administered steroids both in low and high doses. A multicentre trial comparing both dose regimes failed to demonstrate any statistically significant improvement (Collins 1983; Bracken *et al.* 1984, 1985). A randomized controlled trial of methyl prednisolone, naloxone, and placebo (Bracken *et al.* 1990) suggested, however, statistically significant neurological improvement with high doses of methyl prednisolone administered within 8 hours from injury. Information about the size of the population who improved and the degree of improvement, i.e. whether a small number of patients improved significantly or a large number of patients showed little improvement; information about whether it was improvement of density or level, or whether the improvement was local or distal, and the number of patients with Brown-Séquard Syndrome in each group all require consideration in the evaluation of the clinical significance of the statistics.

The advocates of surgical decompression believe that mechanical compression by bony fragment and/or soft tissue is likely to be responsible for some of the persistent neurological deficit, especially in patients with incomplete spinal cord injury. Complete anatomical transection of the spinal cord is rare (Bohlman 1979). Of 67 patients who had a clinically complete injury, 50 showed some continuity across the injured segments (Kakulas 1988).

Whether it is possible to halt or reverse the secondary injury by early decompression is still unclear in the clinical situation.

Pathophysiology of spinal cord injury

The macro- and microscopic pathology of spinal cord injuries has been well described by Hughes (1978). The area of interest in the traumatized spinal cord is centred around the microvascular circulation (Turnbull 1971; White 1975). Of note is the absence of any interconnection of the terminal arteries in the spinal cord, though there is an extensive network of interlocking capillaries around the cord (Turnbull 1971). The capillaries are significantly increased in the central grey matter to accommodate the increased metabolic demand in this area, to the extent that each neuron is connected to at least one capillary.

Understanding the spinal cord blood-flow will lead to the realization that extraspinal circulatory changes are very likely to affect the injured cord. Korbine *et al.* (1975) reported loss of autoregulation in the lateral columns of the traumatized cord. As such the cardio-vascular status and haemoglobin with its oxygen-carrying capacity must not be seen as unrelated or isolated. Turnbull (1971), Ducker and Perot (1971), Assenmacher and Ducker (1971), Ducker *et al.* (1971), Dohrmann *et al.* (1971, 1973) and White *et al.* (1969) have indicated that the microvascular changes following a spinal cord injury are reflected initially in the grey matter, and that there is a correlation between the neurological deficit and the degree of subsequent involvement of the white matter. The biochemical changes at the site of impact also correlate with the vascular status in that the cord oxygen drops almost immediately at the site of the traumatized segment, as noticed in the dog (Kelly *et al.* 1970, 1972). Ducker and Perot (1971) confirmed this but found that it occurs between 2 and 3 hours after the injury. It is preceded by a reduction in blood-flow.

Within about $1\frac{1}{2}$ minutes a significant rise in the lactate levels lasting for about 24 hours was observed by Locke *et al.* (1971). By 1 hour after injury multiple areas of haemorrhage are present in the central grey matter, with generalized loss of cellular architecture in the grey matter. This is followed by the coalescence of the micro-haemorrhages within the grey matter at 2–4 hours following the injury (White *et al.* 1969).

An increase in the water content of the spinal cord appears as early as 5 minutes after trauma, and persists for as long as 15 days (Yashon *et al.* 1973). It is clear that there are a number of parameters that can be measured in the experimental situation, though with some difficulty. Different experimental treatment regimes have been undertaken in the hope of manipulating these parameters. As yet a correlation between the efficiency of this manipulation and its neurological outcome in the laboratory with events in the clinical situation remains to be proven.

Problems of the experimental model

Osterholm (1978) highlighted the difficulties encountered with the reproducibility of results in the controlled laboratory environment. The experiments of Allen in 1911 suggested that the rapidity of the initial insult has a significant bearing on the outcome of cord injury. Slow compression irrespective of size may give rise to minimal neurological fall-out. A small acute compression, however, has a profound effect, frequently causing complete cell destruction. Olsson (1971) and Dohrmann and Panjabi (1976) demonstrated that by dropping different weights from different heights to achieve a 400 gm/cm impact on the cat spinal cord, using an impounder, the volume of the lesion produced in the spinal cord was variable despite the controlled experimental design.

They demonstrated that the amount of energy transferred to the spinal cord was dependent upon factors such as height, impounder mass, and velocity. The latter authors in 1978 also stated that 'force may well be a most reasonable means of quantitating experimental spinal cord trauma'. These factors are virtually impossible to measure in the clinical situation. To date there are no investigative procedures to measure accurately the initial volume of the spinal cord lesion. The previous factors can explain the difficulties in comparing outcome of different management procedures and producing convincing statistical evidence for the superiority of one method of management over others.

Improvement following spinal surgical decompression is currently suggested in various experimental studies. In Bohlman and colleagues' (1979) study of anterior screw compression on the spinal cord of dogs, it is noteworthy that all animals became paralysed to varying degrees. However, despite the ongoing compression some began to improve their cord function. Of the eight dogs with piston compression, three did not require any decompressive surgery to regain their pre-operative neurological status. Although the remaining five animals required decompression to recover, their pre-operative neurological status is not revealed.

Dolan et al. (1980) used the clip compression model, with forces ranging from 16 gm–178 gm and duration of compression ranging from 3 seconds to 900 seconds, in four different groups of rats. They suggest that following decompression, the subsequent functional recovery over a period of 8 weeks was related to the duration of compression regardless of the actual force. Among the difficulties in extrapolating this to the human situation is the fact that the latest decompression in the experimental model was done 15 minutes after compression.

The same laboratory in 1987 (Guha et al. 1987) used the same injury model but with a smaller range of forces applied to the cord. These forces ranged between 2.3 and 53.0 gm, and decompression was performed after 15, 60, 120, and 240 minutes of compression. Functional recovery was assessed weekly for 8 weeks. They found that animals injured with the low forces (2.3 gm clips) performed significantly better than those injured with higher forces for all times until decompression. There was also a significant difference in recovery between the groups injured by the 16.9 and 53.0 gm clips, although only for the group decompressed at 15 minutes. Early decompression did not improve the neurological outcome with the 53 gm clip. The animals compressed at 2.3 gm and decompressed after 15 or 16 minutes had significantly better function than those decompressed after long periods (120–240 minutes).

The authors concluded that, with lower forces, decompression as early as possible and within 240 minutes (simulating the clinical situation) can be beneficial.

We feel that, apart from the control group of rats whose spinal cords were not compressed the inclusion of another group of rats with unrelieved compression might have helped to simulate the clinical situation with its attendant controversy. The neurological outcome of rats with unrelieved compression, especially of the lower magnitude, would have been most interesting to observe.

Decompression by establishing anatomical reduction

Most clinicians would agree that reduction and restoration of vertebral alignment is accompanied by some decompression of the spinal cord (Jacobs and Casey 1984; Dickson *et al.* 1978; Yosipovitch *et al.* 1977; Fletsch *et al.* 1977; White *et al.* 1980).

Wiberg and Hauge (1988) found that decompression was not always achieved following the application of distraction rods and realignment of the spine in thoracic and lumbar injuries. On re-exploration of the ventral aspect of the spinal canal, there was significant compression from bone fragments in 43 per cent of patients in the latter study. McAFee *et al.* (1985) and Jelsma *et al.* (1982) reported similar cases where following restoration of alignment by distraction rods there was persistent compression.

Frankel *et al.* (1969) found no correlation between the bony lesions, the various degrees of reduction, and the neurological lesion. Durward *et al.* (1981) observed poor correlation between the degree of canal compromise as measured by computerized tomography and the resulting neurological deficit.

The following case history demonstrates that reduction is not imperative for the achievement of neurological improvement. The value of conservative management is postulated:

A 74-year-old lady was involved in a road-traffic accident at the age of 60. She sustained a bilateral facet dislocation of C5 upon C6 as well as a fracture of the pedicle of C2. The initial clinical presentation indicated a symmetrical weakness of the wrist extensors and the triceps, with minimal power in the intrinsic muscles of the hand. There was no power in the lower extremities; no control of the bladder or bowel, but complete sensory preservation. Her reflexes in the biceps and triceps were present, but absent in the lower limbs.

The patient was managed in skull traction without effectively reducing the cervical dislocation. Despite this she began to recover function to the lower limbs and the hands at 2 days. Skull traction was discontinued at 6 weeks. At 3 months after the injury the patient was walking and demonstrated control of her bowel and bladder.

After 13 years the patient had full power in the legs, with hyperreflexia of the lower limbs. The only deficit was confined to the left hand, which demonstrated minimal loss of full wrist extensor power [4/5] and the loss of power of the intrinsic muscles of the hand, which did not recover.

The first X-ray demonstrates the fracture of the pedicle of C2 and bilateral dislocation of the facets at C5/C6 (Fig. 1.1). The second X-ray (10 years after the injury) confirms the union of the above injury, still in the dislocated position (Fig. 1.2).

In our experience late reduction of the cervical spine (after 48 hours) can result in a significant neurological deterioration. We believe that it is particularly hazardous for the inexperienced clinician to attempt closed reduction at this late stage.

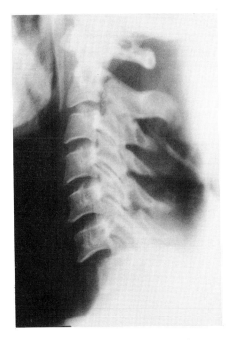

Fig. 1.1. Lateral radiograph of the cervical spine with a fracture of the pedicle in C2, and a bilateral dislocation of the facet joints C6 upon C7.

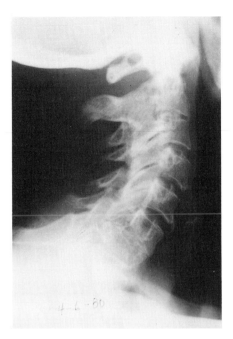

Fig. 1.2. Lateral radiograph of the cervical spine ten years later. Follow-up demonstrating the healed pedicle fracture of C2 and the union of C6 to C7 in the dislocated position.

The current difficulty in predicting which type of injury will benefit from decompression by establishing anatomical reduction is probably due to the fact that the commonly available diagnostic tools do not allow complete and exact identification of the details of the injury. It may be that bony fragments attached to the undamaged posterior longitudinal ligament encroaching on the canal and/or spinal cord would be stretched away from the canal and its contents by distraction/reduction. In this instance, establishing anatomical alignment would be beneficial. If, however, the posterior longitudinal ligament is torn or the bony fragment is not attached to this ligament, reduction or retraction are unlikely to be accompanied by decompression. Another cause of failure of the decompression is 'locking' of the bony fragments. Further work with Magnetic Resonance Imaging (MRI), with its capacity to delineate ligaments, may contribute to the identification of those injuries in which decompression is likely to succeed with distraction and or realignment (see Figs. 1.3, 1.4, and 1.5).

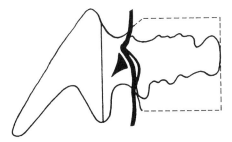

Fig. 1.3. Sagittal section of the vertebral body indicating the bony fragment separate from the posterior longitudinal ligament, precluding it from effective reduction by distraction.

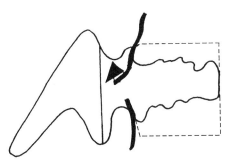

Fig. 1.4. Sagittal section through the vertebral body demonstrating a torn posterior longitudinal ligament and its inability to produce reduction despite traction.

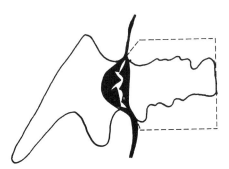

Fig. 1.5. Sagittal section through the vertebral body showing 'locking' of the bony fragments, which in turn prevent complete reduction despite traction.

Decompression by laminectomy

Routine decompressive laminectomy has little to offer to patients with spinal injury (Seljeskog 1982; Wiberg and Hauge 1988; McAFee *et al.* 1985). Furthermore it can lead to and/or increase instability and spinal deformity (Verbiest 1963; Jacobs and Casey 1984; Bradford *et al.* 1977; Bohlman and Eismont 1981; McAFee *et al.* 1985).

Neurological deterioration following laminectomy was highlighted by Guttmann (1949), Benassy *et al.* (1967), Morgan *et al.* (1971), Bohlman (1979), and Dickson *et al.* (1978).

In the presence of the narrowed spinal canal and an injured spinal cord the jaws of the rongeur removing the laminae can inflict further damage to the cord (Verbiest 1963). Adequate decompression cannot be achieved by laminectomy when the compressive element is in the anterior aspect of the canal (Bradford *et al.* 1977; Fleisch *et al.* 1977). Laminectomies are still done in conjunction with other surgical procedures such as posterior instrumentation (Seljeskog 1982) and pedicular screwing of the Roy-Camille's plate, (Lagarrigue *et al.* 1980).

Our indication for laminectomy is empirically restricted to patients who may deteriorate with an ascending neurological deficit of more than 2–3 segments, when computerized tomography reveals posterior compression of the spinal cord or cauda equina by bony fragments or soft tissue. This is however a rather infrequent occurrence.

Anterior decompression

During this last decade we have seen enthusiasm in some surgical quarters for decompression of the anterior aspect of the spinal canal through an anterior approach or a postero-lateral approach, depending on the level and the type of injury. This is possibly related to the disappointing results of routine laminectomy, the lack of convincing evidence that surgical realignment and internal fixation improved the neurological outcome, the possible neurological deterioration with sublaminar wiring (Rossier and Cochran 1984), and the advent of computerized tomography, revealing anterior compression of the neural tissue as well as narrowing of the sagittal diameter of the canal. The proponents of anterior decompression believe that in patients with an incomplete neurological lesion, improvement can be achieved by the surgical removal of the elements encroaching on the canal. This is suggested as a treatment modality for the cervical spine by Bohlman and Eismont (1981), and in the dorso-lumbar spine by Kadena *et al.* (1984), McAFee *et al.* (1985), McEvoy and Bradford (1985), and Dunn (1986). Indeed further collapse of the vertebral column has been observed by Gertzbein *et al.* (1988) following anterior decompression. A further surgical stabilizing procedure is usually necessary in view of the additional instability that could occur. Dislodging of an anterior bony graft has been observed by the authors in the cervical spine following decompression without stabilization.

While it is possible to combine anterior decompression with posterior stabilization and fusion or anterior plating, in a one-stage procedure, this is likely to be associated with increased mortality and morbidity if contemplated within the first 50 hours from injury in a patient with a multi-system deficit.

Decompression is usually performed at the site of the vertebral fracture or fracture dislocation. Assenmacher and Ducker (1971) demonstrated that in an experimental traumatic paraplegia the vascular and pathological changes seen in irreversible cord lesions can extend up to 5 times the length of the traumatized segment. Indeed in the two post-mortem specimens we examined following the death of two patients with complete spinal cord injuries, the cord lesion did extend beyond the traumatized unit of motion. It was argued that in these two patients anterior decompression restricted to the site of the fracture would have been incomplete. The incidence of this problem is not yet known. Furthermore we are in agreement with Bedbrook (1975, 1979) that early myelography is of no clinical value in distinguishing the extent of damage in the spinal cord, nor of management value, in determining the need for decompression (Guttmann 1973). It might be possible in the near future to determine the volume and the extent of the cord lesion by MRI imaging and spectroscopy.

Myelotomy

Allen in 1911 reported that in dogs with severe cord injury, death would occur unless myelotomy was performed. Freeman and Wright (1953) performed myelotomy following experimental spinal injuries on dogs, and reported better than expected neurological improvement compared to the untreated animals.

The beneficial effects of myelotomy may be explained by a number of possible mechanisms. The removal of pressure, blood, and necrotic tissue from within the spinal cord has been postulated by Allen (1914) and Campbell *et al.* (1973); by decreasing cavitation, thus protecting the surviving axons from further damage (Freeman and Wright 1953), or by improving spinal cord blood-flow from the reduction in tissue pressure and vasoactive substances (Rivlin and Tator 1979). However the procedure could cause irreversible cord damage (Scarff 1960) or some further destruction of cord tissue (Tarlov 1957). Benes in 1968 performed myelotomy in 20 patients, four of whom were eventually able to walk with crutches. Unfortunately the completeness of the lesion prior to surgery could not be ascertained. The death-rate following the procedure was 40 per cent.

Although we have no direct experience with the procedure we know of cases where 'toothpaste-like' cord material had exuded through dural tear during surgical decompression. We are not aware of any surgeon undertaking this procedure routinely in the present time.

Timing of surgical decompression

There is no general agreement between surgeons as to the optimum timing of surgical decompression by whichever method. Immediate or early decompression is advocated by Bedoiseau et al. (1971), Jacobs (1980), and Dunn (1986).

Wiberg and Hauge (1988) believe that early surgery may have been beneficial, with neurological improvement, in two of his patients who presented with complete cord injuries and who were decompressed within 10 hours after the accident.

On the other hand Larson et al. (1976), McAFee et al. (1985), Bedbrook (1975, 1979), Bradford et al. (1977), and Willen et al. (1985) believe that early or immediate surgical decompression does not appear to provide additional neurological recovery in the severely contused spine.

By comparing the neurological outcome of patients with cauda equina lesions who had undergone immediate, early, and late decompression, Fleisch et al. (1977) could not show any difference in the neurological recovery.

It is difficult to determine the value of early decompression in view of the dynamic nature of the neurological picture. It is a well-known fact that a certain degree of spontaneous neurological recovery occurs in many patients with incomplete neurological lesions and in some patients with complete paralysis on presentation. Furthermore, neurological deterioration associated with active intervention cannot be measured or ruled out.

Complications of surgical decompression and conservative management

The injured swollen cord is probably especially vulnerable to any further trauma, however minimal. Rossier and Cochran (1984) reported deterioration in a patient with dorsal injury and another patient with dorso-lumbar injury, following open reduction and sublaminar wiring with Harrington compression rods. Wiberg and Hauge (1988) reported cord swelling during surgical decompression converting incomplete (subtotal) lesions into complete lesions. They reported protrusion of 'oedematous cord substance ... like toothpaste through dural rents'. Transient neurological deterioration was also observed immediately following surgery in 'several cases' undergoing an anterior decompression and/or a posterior procedure by Gertzbein et al. (1988). McAFee et al. (1985) reported on 70 patients with spinal cord injury and dorso-lumbar fractures treated by anterior spinal cord decompression: three of these cases had transient neurological deterioration from radiculopathy; while Bohlman and Eismont (1981) reported three patients who deteriorated following post-operative improvement in a series of 100 patients who had undergone late decompression of the cervical spine.

Dunn (1986) states that significant complications occur following anterior stabilization and decompression for thoraco-lumbar injuries. He feels, however, that on balance the neurological recovery of his patients with incomplete lesions was more favourable than those of the Frankel *et al.* (1969) and the Dickson *et al.* (1978) series.

Non-neurological complications such as pneumonia, respiratory distress, pulmonary compromise, oesophageal perforation, thoracic duct tear, graft extrusion, and graft collapse have been reported in the literature following surgery, as well as meningitis and brain damage.

With conservative management and frequent, regular, accurate neurological examination we have observed in a small number of patients a transient ascent of the neurological level involving one or two segments above the level of the lesion. This usually occurs within 48–120 hours following the injury. This is almost invariably temporary, and we confirm the observation by Frankel (1969) that within a few weeks the initial neurological level descends to correspond to that found immediately following the injury, or even to a lower level.

A less common form of deterioration, with permanent ascent in the level of lesion of more than 2 segments and up to 7 segments, occurs in about 1.5 per cent of patients with mainly dorso-lumbar injuries, usually within the first two weeks following the injury and less commonly in the third week following the accident (Frankel 1969). The pathology of this condition is not clear, however: the final neurological outcome in six out of the seven patients documented by Frankel was flaccid paralysis, suggesting a vascular aetiology. The one patient who had two laminectomies performed did not improve. The incidence of transient neurological ascent of 1 or 2 levels of lesion is not well documented in the operative management series. The topography extent, and type of paralysis when deterioration occurs following surgery is not usually well described. Indeed it may be difficult to determine post-operatively if a neurological deterioration is due to the natural injury process or is related in someway to the surgical procedure (Stauffer 1989).

When approaching the management of spinal injury one needs to consider the 'spinal cord instability' as well as the vertebral column instability. In the unstable vertebral injury there is a potential risk for further displacement and mechanical compression on the spinal cord resulting in further neurological deterioration. This instabilty is usually contained by either conservative or surgical means. Neurological deterioration can occur, however, owing to factors unrelated to mechanical compression. The pathophysiological changes in the spinal cord suggest the presence of an inherent physiological instability following trauma (El Masri *et al.*, in press). Indeed hypotension, hypothermia, hypoxia, or septicaemia can result in neurological deterioration or slow down the neurological recovery rate in patients with incomplete lesions.

This association has been observed by us as well as by clinicians from both the conservative and the surgical schools. The effect of anaesthetic agents on the traumatized spinal cord requires thorough assessment.

Patients with spinal cord injury initially have a multi-system deficit which can be the source of many complications, and may result in hypotension, hypoxia, and infections. Anaesthetic and/or surgical procedures can, at least potentially, increase the risk of these complications. Whether extreme care would completely abolish the extra risk of neurological deterioration is arguable.

Neurological outcome of management

To date there is no convincing evidence that the final neurological outcome is favourably altered by surgical decompression. Young and Dexter (1978) found no statistically significant difference between the neurological progression of their patients and those reported in the earlier Stoke Mandeville study by Frankel *et al.* (1969). We have found no convincing evidence of any advantageous neurological outcome following surgery by carefully analysing McAFee and colleagues' series (1985) of anterior decompression for thoraco-lumbar fractures with incomplete neurological deficit; Wiberg's and Hauge's series (1988) of surgery for the thoracic and lumbar spine treated with Harrington distraction device and additional anterior decompression in 43 per cent of patients; or the Gertzbein *et al.* series of 1988. The last also concluded that there was no clear difference in the outcome between anterior versus posterior surgery, regardless of the level of the lesion. Osti *et al.* (1989) reviewed their patients with cervical injuries and concluded that early surgical stabilization of the cervical spine using a dowel interbody fusion seemed to impair neurological recovery in patients with neurological deficit. Tator *et al.* (1987) compared the outcome of surgical and conservative management in 208 patients with acute spinal cord injury. They have shown that statistically there was no difference between operated and non-surgically treated patients in length of stay or in neurological recovery. Wilmot and Hall (1986) found no difference in the neurological outcome between surgically and conservatively treated patients with paraplegia.

Folman and El Masri (1989) reviewed 70 patients with closed traumatic incomplete injuries of the spinal cord admitted within 72 hours of their accident to the Midland Centre for Spinal Injuries, and treated conservatively.

There were 50 patients with incomplete cervical and 20 patients with incomplete thoracic cord injuries. No patients with cauda equina or root lesions were included. The Frankel classification was used for an average follow-up of 4.7 years. Of the 37 patients who presented with sensory sparing only (group B) 24 patients [65 per cent] recovered useful motor function, of whom 5 patients made full recovery. Of the 21 patients presenting with useless motor sparing (group C) 18 patients [86 per cent] recovered useful motor function, of whom 12 [60 per cent] recovered completely. Of the 12 patients who presented with useful motor sparing (group D) 9 patients [75 per cent] recovered completely. Gotfried and El Masri are presently reviewing a series of patients with dorso-lumbar lesions treated conservatively. Our impression is that patients with cauda equina lesions have an even better neurological outcome than patients with cord lesions, and that the results of conservative management compare favourably with surgical decompression.

The following case history highlights the value of conservative management of the dorso-lumbar fracture with a cauda equina lesion:

JS, a 19-year-old girl, was involved in a motor-cycle accident on 1/8/87. She presented a burst fracture of the first lumbar vertebra. Her clinical picture demonstrated weakness of the lower limbs, with a symmetrical loss of power in the hip muscles of grade 2/5 and a power of 2/5 in the rest of the lower limb. The knee and ankle reflexes were absent on admission. She had analgesia to pinprick in the S1 to S5 areas bilaterally, and no bladder or bowel control. Her initial X-rays demonstrate the burst fracture of L1, and the CAT scan confirms the retropulsion of fragments into the canal, almost obliterating it.

The patient was treated conservatively with bed-rest for a period of 6 weeks, and at that time her power in the legs had improved to grade 4/5 throughout and the sensory deficit had improved in the S3 dermatome. During this period the S3–S5 dermatome was still analgesic to pinprick, and the bladder and bowels required manual expression.

At about three months after the accident the patient had regained her bladder function as well as a partial return of sensation in the sacral dermatomes.

At the two-year follow-up the patient is able to walk as far as she wants and the power in the legs is normal. She still has a diminished sensory perception to pinprick in the sacral segments, but her bladder and bowel control is normal. Both the knee and the ankle reflexes have returned. She demonstrates improvement despite the ongoing neural compression. The range of movement in her dorso-lumbar spine is normal (Figs. 1.6, 1.7, and 1.8).

There is concern amongst some clinicians that bony fragments left unremoved in the spinal canal may produce further neurological deterioration either in the short or the long term. This is not borne out by our own experience. Evidence of remodelling of the spinal canal with receding of the bony fragments has been reported recently by Weinstein *et al.* (1988) and Fidler (1988). The recession or disappearance of the bony fragment from the canal in some cases may explain why late neurological deterioration, other than that due to post-traumatic syringomyelia, is most unlikely to happen, especially in the cauda equina lesions.

Most studies attempting to define the place of surgery in the management of spinal cord injured patients have compared a group of patients treated by a single method with either a historical control group from the same institution or from the literature treated by another method (Tator *et al.* 1987). Although prospective randomized controlled studies would be of value in determining the benefits of any surgical procedure including late decompression, there are a number of problems which may explain why such a study has not been done. The multitude of patterns of injuries and of the opinions for the treatment of any particular injury, the dynamic nature of the pathology and the clinical neurological progression, the difficulty of accurate assessment of the rate of the neurological progress, the variable times of presentation of the patient with spinal cord injury to the specialist units, the different emphasis on the importance of certain medications, the lack of an easy objective method for prospective evaluation, the unavailability of accurate investigative diagnostic procedures, the poor resources in some specialist units, and the need for several specialized centres to co-operate in such a study are some of the reasons why it has not yet been done. This is not to say that it is beyond the ingenuity of our caring profession.

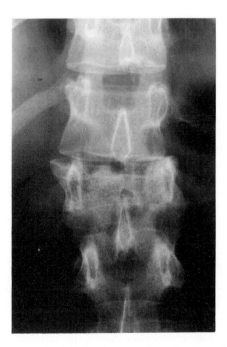

Fig. 1.6. Anterior radiograph of the lumbar vertebrae showing a burst fracture of L1.

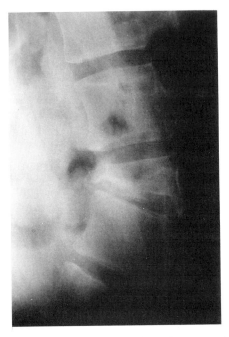

Fig. 1.7. Lateral radiograph of the lumbar vertebrae demonstrating the burst fracture of L1.

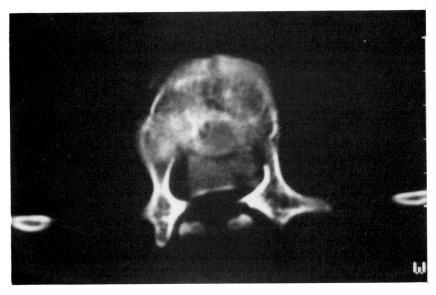

Fig. 1.8. CAT scan of the L1 vertebra showing the retropulsion of the 'body' of L1 almost obliterating the canal.

Conclusions

Early surgical decompression has yet to prove particularly beneficial to the neurological outcome of patients with spinal cord injury. In our experience the great majority of patients presenting with sensory or motor sparing as early as 6 hours following the injury or later will make some neurological recovery with conservative management. In general the more neurological sparing is evident at presentation, the greater the degree of expected recovery. Recovery is likely to continue for about 18 months following the injury; however, the rate of the recovery is usually much higher in the first 6 months. During the first 2 months following injury, the spinal cord is physiologically unstable and vulnerable to hypoxia, hypotension, hypothermia, and septicaemia. Anaesthesia and surgery present an extra potential hazard to the injured cord in inexperienced hands. To date we have reserved decompression for the occasional patient who may show significant neurological deterioration. However, we have no evidence of its beneficial value. We feel that MRI imaging and spectroscopy, when refined, are likely to contribute to our understanding of the pathological processes in the spinal cord, and may help us improve our understanding of the role of early decompression in the management of spinal cord injury. We would be prepared to consider early surgical decompression if and when objective evidence of its beneficial value becomes available.

References

Allen, A. R. (1911). Surgery of experimental lesion of spinal cord equivalent to crush injury or fracture dislocation of spinal column. A preliminary report. *Journal of the American Medical Association*, **57**, 878–80.

Allen, A. R. (1914). Remarks on the histopathological changes in the spinal cord due to impact. An experimental study. *Journal of Nervous and Mental Disease*, **41**, 141–7.

Assenmacher, D. R. and Ducker, T. B. (1971). Experimental traumatic paraplegia; the vascular and pathological changes seen in reversible and irreversible cord lesions. *Journal of Bone and Joint Surgery*, **53A**, 671–80.

Bedbrook, G. M. (1969). Use and disuse of surgery in the lumbar-dorso fractures. *Journal of the Western Pacific Orthopaedic Association*, **6**, 5–26.

Bedbrook, G. M. (1975). Treatment of thoracolumbar dislocation and fractures with paraplegia. *Clinical Orthopaedics*, **112**, 27–43.

Bedbrook, G. M. (1979). Spinal injuries with tetraplegia and paraplegia. *Journal of Bone and Joint Surgery*, **61B**, 267–84.

Bedoiseau, M., Roy Carville, R., Roy Carmille, M., and Saillant, G. (1971). Examen clinique d'un traumatisé récent de la moelle. Conclusions prognostiques et therapeutiques immédiates. *Revue pratique*, **21**(25), 3707–28.

Benassy, J., Blauchand, J., and Lecoq, P. (1967). Neurological recovery rate in paraplegia and tetraplegia. *Paraplegia*, **4**, 259–69.

Benes, V. (1968). *Spinal cord injury*, pp. 94–6. Baillière, London.

Bohlman, H. H. (1979). Acute fractures and dislocations of the cervical spine. *Journal of Bone and Joint Surgery*, **61A**, 1119–42.

Bohlman, H. H. and Eismont, F. J. (1981). Surgical techniques of anterior decompression and fusion for spinal cord injuries. *Clinical Orthopaedics*, **54**, 57–67.

Bracken, M. B., Collins, W. F., Freeman, D. F., Shephard, M. J., Wagner, F. W., Silten, R. M., *et al.* (1984). Efficacy of methyl prednisolone in acute spinal cord injury. *Journal of the American Medical Association*, **251**, 45–57.

Bracken, M. B., Shepard, M. J., and Hellebrand, K. G. (1985). Methyl prednisolone and neurological function 1 year after spinal cord injury (National acute spinal cord injury study). *Journal of Neurosurgery*, **63**, 704–13.

Bracken, M. B., Shepard, M. J., Collins, W. F., Holford, T. R., Young, W., Baskin, D. S., *et al.* (1990). A randomized controlled trial of methylprednisolone or naloxone in the treatment of acute spinal-cord injury: results of the Second National Acute Spinal Cord Injury Study. *New England Journal of Medicine*, **322**, 1405–11.

Bradford, D. S., Akbarnia, B. A., Winter, R. B., and Selgeskog, E. L. (1977). Surgical stabilization of fracture and fracture dislocations of the thoracic spine. *Spine*, **2**, 185–96.

Burke, D. C., Duncan, M., and Scotia, N. (1976). The management of thoracic and thoracolumbar injuries of the spine with neurological involvement. *Journal of Bone and Joint Surgery*, **58B**, 72–8.

Campbell, J. B., Decrescito, V., Tomasula, J. J., Demopoulos, H. B., Flamm, E. S., and Ransohoff, J. (1973). Experimental spinal cord contusion in the cat. *Journal of Surgical Neurology*, **1**, 102–6.

Collins, W. F. (1983). A review and update of experiment and clinical studies of spinal cord injury. *Paraplegia*, **21**, 204–19.

Dickson, J. H., Harrington, P. R., and Ewin, W. D. (1978). Results of reduction and stabilisation of the severely fractured thoracic and lumbar spine. *Journal of Bone and Joint Surgery*, **60A**, 799–805.

Dolan, E. G., Tator, C. H., and Endrenyl, L. (1980). The value of decompression of acute experimental spinal cord compression. *Journal of Neurosurgery*, **53**, 749–55.

Dohrmann, G. J. and Panjabi, M. M. (1976). 'Standardised' spinal cord trauma. Biochemical parameters and lesion volume. *Surgical Neurology*, **6**, 263–76.

Dohrmann, G. J. and Panjabi, M. M. (1978). Biomechanics of experimental spinal cord trauma. *Journal of Neurosurgery*, **48**, 993–1001.

Dohrmann, G. J., Wagner, F. L., and Bucy, P. C. (1971). The microvasculature in the transistory traumatic paraplegic. An electron microscopic study in the Moubey. *Journal of Neurosurgery*, **35**, 263–71.

Dohrmann, G. J., Wich, K., and Bucy, P. C. (1973). Spinal cord blood flow patterns in experimental traumatic paraplegia. *Journal of Neurosurgery*, **38**, 52–8.

Ducker, T. B. and Hamit, H. F. (1969). Experimental treatment of acute spinal cord injury. *Journal of Neurosurgery*, **30**, 693–7.

Ducker, T. B. and Perot, P. L. (1971). Spinal cord blood flow and oxygen in trauma. *Journal of Neurosurgery*, **22**, 413–15.

Ducker, T. B., Kindt, G. W., and Kempe, L. G. (1971). Pathological findings in acute and experimental cord trauma. *Journal of Neurosurgery*, **35**, 700–8.

Dunn, H. K. (1986). Anterior spine stabilisation and decompression for thoracolumbar injuries. *Orthopaedic Clinics of North America*, **17**(1), 113–19.

Durward, R. J., Schweigel, J. F., and Harrison, P. (1981). Management of fractures of the thoraco lumbar and lumbar spine. *Journal of Neurosurgery*, **8**, 555–61.

El Masri, W. S., Baker, H. J., Pringle, R. G., and Frankel, H. L. Physiological instability of the spinal cord following injury. (In press.)

Fidler, M. W. (1988). Remodeling of the spinal canal after burst fracture. *Journal of Bone and Joint Surgery*, **70B**, 730–2.

Fleisch, J. R., Leiden, L. L., Erickson, D. L., Chou, S. N., and Bradford, D. S. (1977). Harrington instrumentation and spinal fusion for unstable fractures and fracture dislocations of the thoracic and lumbar spine. *Journal of Bone and Joint Surgery*, **59A**, 143–53.

Folman, Y. and El Masri, W. S. (1989). Spinal cord injury prognostic indicators. *Injury*, **20**, 92–3.

Frankel, H. L. (1969). Ascending cord lesion in the early stages following spinal injury. *Paraplegia*, **7**, 111–18.

Frankel, H. L., Hankock, D. O., Hyslop, G., Helzak, J., Michealis, L. S., Ungar, G. H., *et al.* (1969). The value of postural reduction in the initial management of closed injuries of the spine with paraplegia and tetraplegia. *Paraplegia*, **7**, 179–92.

Freeman, L. W. and Wright, T. W. (1953). Experimental observations of concussion and contusion of the spinal cord. *Annals of Surgery*, **137**, 433–43.

Gertzbein, S. D., Count-Brown, C. M., Marks, P., Martin, C., Fazl, M., Schwartz,M., *et al.* (1988). The neurological outcome following surgery of spinal fractures. *Spine*, **13**, 641–4.

Guha, A., Tator, C. H., Endreyl, L., and Piper, I. (1987). Decompression of the spinal cord improves recovery after acute experimental spinal cord compression injury. *Praplegia*, **25**, 324–39.

Guttmann, L. (1949). Surgical aspects of treatment of traumatic paraplegia. *Journal of Bone and Joint Surgery*, **31B**, 399–403.

Guttmann, L. (1973). *Spinal cord injuries. Comprehensive management and research*, p. 137. Blackwell Scientific Publications, Oxford.

Guttmann, L. (1976). *Spinal cord injuries. Comprehensive management and research*. (2nd edn), pp. 142–51. Blackwell Scientific Publications, Oxford.

Hughes, T. J. (1978). *Pathology of the spinal cord* (2nd edn). Lloyd-Luke, London.

Jacobs, R., Asher, M. A., and Snider, R. K. (1980). Thoraco-lumbar spinal injuries. A comparative study of recumbent and operative treatment in 100 patients. *Spine*, **5**, 463–77.

Jacobs, R. R. and Casey, M. P. (1984). Surgical management of the thoraco-lumbar spinal injuries. *Clinical Orthopaedics*, **189**, 22–35.

Jelsma, R. K., Kisslh, P. T., Jelsme, L. F., Ramsey, W. L., and Rice, J. F. (1982). Surgical treatment of the thoraco-lumbar fractures. *Surgical Neurology*, **18**, 156–66.

Kadena, K., Abumi, K., and Fugiya, M. (1984). Burst fracture with neurological deficit of the thoraco-lumbar spine. Results of decompression and stabilisation with anterior instrumentation. *Spine*, **9**, 788–95.

Kakulas, A. (1988). The applied neurobiology of human spinal cord injury: a review. *Paraplegia*, **26**, 371–9.

Kelly, D. L., Lassiter, K. R., Calogero, J. A., and Alexander, E. (jun.) (1970). Effects of local hypothermia and tissue oxygen studies in experimental paraplegia. *Journal of Neurosurgery*, **33**, 554–63.

Kelly, D. L., Lassiter, K. R., Vongsvivret, V., and Smith, J. H. (1972). Effects of hyperbaric oxygenation and tissue oxygen studies in experimental paraplegia. *Journal of Neurosurgery*, **36**, 425–9.

Korbine, A. I., Doyle, T. F., and Martins, A. N. (1975). Local spinal cord blood flow in experimental traumatic myelopathy. *Journal of Neurosurgery*, **42**, 144–9.

Lagarrigue, J., Lazother, Y., Zadeh, J. D., Verdie, J. C., Richaud, J., and Chaput, J. P. (1980). Traitement par plaques vissées de Roy-Camille des fractures graves du rachis dorsal et lombaire. *Revue de médecine de Toulouse*, **XVI**, 99–107.

Larson, S. J., Holst, R. A., Hemmy, D. C., and Sanch, A. (jun.) (1976). Lateral extracavity approach to traumatic lesions of the thoracic and lumbar spine. *Journal of Neurosurgery*, **45**, 628–37.

Lewis, J. and McKibbin, B. (1974). The treatment of unstable fracture dislocation of the thoraco-lumbar spine accompanied by paraplegia. *Journal of Bone and Joint Surgery*, **56B**, 603–12.

Locke, G. E., Yashon, D., Feldman, R. A., and Hunt, W. E. (1971). Ischaemic in primate spinal cord injury. *Journal of Neurosurgery*, **34**, 614–17.

McAFee, P. C., Bohlmann, H. H., and Yuan, H. A. (1985). Anterior decompression of traumatic thoraco-lumbar fractures with incomplete neurological deficit using a retroperitoneal approach. *Journal of Bone and Joint Surgery*, **67A**, 89–104.

McEvoy, R. D. and Bradford, D. S. (1985). The management of burst fractures of the thoracic and lumbar spine. Experience in 53 patients. *Spine*, **10**, 631–7.

Morgan, T. H., Wharton, G. W., and Austin, G. N. (1971). The result of laminectomy in patients with incomplete spinal cord injuries. *Paraplegia*, **9**, 14–23.

Olsson, Sten-Eric (1971). The dynamic factor in spinal cord compression. *Journal of Neurosurgery*, **35**, 308–20.

Osterholm, J.L. (1978). *The pathology of spinal cord trauma*, American Lecture Series. Charles C. Thomas, Springfield, Illinois.

Osti, O. L., Fraser, R. D., and Griffith, E. R. (1989). Reduction and stabilisation of cervical dislocations. An analysis of 167 cases. *Journal of Bone and Joint Surgery*, **71B**, 275–82.

Rivlin, A. S. and Tator, C. H. (1979). Effect of vesodilatus and myclotomy on recovery after acute spinal cord injury in rats. *Journal of Neurosurgery*, **50**, 349–52.

Rossier, A. B. and Cochran, T. P. (1984). The treatment of spinal fractures with Harrington Compression Rods and segmental sublaminar wiring. A dangerous combination. *Spine*, **9**, 796–9.

Scarff, J. E. (1960). Injuries of the vertebral column and spinal cord. In *Injuries of the brain and spinal cord and their coverings* (4th edn) (ed. S. Brock), pp. 530–89. Springer-Verlag, New York.

Seljeskog, E. L. (1982). Thoraco-lumbar injuries. *Clinical Neurosurgery*, **30**, 626–41.

Stauffer, S. (1989). Subaxial injuries. *Clinical Orthopaedics*, **239**, 30–9.

Tarlov, I. M. (1957). *Spinal cord compression. Mechanisms of paralysis and treatment*. Charles C. Thomas, Springfield, Illinois.

Tator, C. H., Duncan, E. G., Edwards, V. E., Lapizak, L. I., and Andrews, D. F. (1987). Comparison of surgical and conservative management in 208 patients with acute spinal cord injury. *Canadian Journal of Neurological Sciences*, **14**, 61–9.

Turnbull, I. (1971). Microvasculature of the human spine cord. *Journal of Neurosurgery*, **35**, 141–6.

Verbiest, H. (1963). Surgery of the cervical vertebral body in cases of traumatic deformity or dislocation. In *Spinal injuries. Proceedings of the symposium* (ed. P. Harris). Royal College of Surgeons of Edinburgh.

Weinstein, J. N., Collalto, P., and Lehmann, T. R. (1988). Thoracolumbar 'burst' fractures treated conservatively: a long term follow up. *Spine*, **13**, 33–8.

White, R. J. (1975). Pathology of the spinal cord in experimental lesions. *Clinical Orthopaedics*, **112**, 16–26.

White, R. J., Albin, M. S., Harris, L. S., and Yasmon, D. (1969). Segmental morphology and hypothermic stabilisation. *Surgical Forum*, **20**, 432.

White, R. J., Newburg, A., and Seligson, D. (1980). Computerised tomographic assessment of the traumatised dorsolumbar spine before and after Harrington instrumentation. *Clinical Orthopaedics*, **146**, 150–6.

Wiberg, J. and Hauge, H. N. (1988). Neurological outcome after surgery for thoracic and lumbar spine injuries. *Acta Neurochirurgica*, **91**, 106–12.

Willen, J., Lindahl, S., and Nordwal, A. (1985). Unstable thoraco-lumbar fractures. A comparative clinical study of conservative treatment and Harrington Instrumentation. *Spine*, **10**, 111–21.

Wilmot, C. B. and Hall, K. M. (1986). Evaluation of acute surgical intervention in traumatic paraplegia. *Paraplegia*, **24**, 71–6.

Yashon, D., Bingham, G. W., Faddoul, E. D. and Hunt, W. E. (1973). Oedema of the spinal cord following experimental trauma. *Journal of Neurosurgery*, **38**, 693–7.

Yosipovitch, Z. U., Robin, G. C., and Myers, M. (1977). Open reduction of unstable thoraco-lumbar spinal injuries and fixation with Harrington Rods. *Journal of Bone and Joint Surgery*, **59A**, 1003–15.

Young, J. S. and Dexter, W. R. (1978). Neurological recovery distal to the zone of injury in 172 cases of closed traumatic spinal cord injury. *Paraplegia*, **16**, 39–49.

2

Therapy of acute spinal cord injury

Wise Young

Introduction

Clinical and laboratory approaches to spinal cord injury maintain the traditional pessimism first expressed in the *Edwin Smith Papyrus* (Breasted 1930), which regarded the possibility of recovery from spinal cord injury as being so remote that it recommended letting spinal-injured warriors die. For example, most clinical categorizations of spinal injury segregate patients into two distinct groups: 'complete' and 'incomplete'. The former are assumed not to recover. Medical care focuses on preservation and protection of peripheral organs, while surgical procedures continue to be oriented towards stabilization of spinal fractures and prevention of further spinal cord injury (Young and Ransohoff 1989). Rehabilitative care of the spinal-injured emphasizes making the best use of residual function. The pessimism has extended to the laboratory, manifested in the assumption by many researchers that regeneration is the only solution to spinal cord injury. This is also reflected in the frequent use of the transected spinal cord for regeneration studies, a preparation designed to eliminate possibilities of spontaneous recovery. The field waits with bated breath for advances in regenerative therapy to restore injured spinal cords.

The acute spinal cord injury response

At the turn of the century Allen (1911, 1914) described an intriguing progression of spinal lesions resulting from dropping a 20 gm weight 20 cm on to exposed thoracic spinal cords. Immediately after the contusion, the injury site shows little histological evidence of tissue damage except for scattered petechial haemorrhages (Goodkin and Campbell 1969). Within several hours, however, gross haemorrhagic necrosis develops in grey matter at the impact site. Lesions in human spinal cords show a similar central haemorrhagic pattern (Spiller 1898; Kakulas and Bedbrook 1969, 1976). Allen's prescient observations did not attract much attention for five decades, until several investigators (Ducker and Assenmacher 1969; Ducker and Perot 1969; Ducker *et al.* 1971; Wagner 1969; Dohrman *et al.* 1973; Osterholm 1974) found evidence of endothelial breakdown and pathological coagulation products in blood-vessels prior to the development of gross necrosis at the lesion site. They and others (Campbell *et al.* 1974; Balentine 1978*a*, *b*; Demopoulos *et al.* 1978) consequently proposed that the endothelial pathology and coagulation in damaged vessels lead to ischaemia and progressive tissue damage at the lesion site.

Blood-flow measurements revealed that grey matter blood-flow falls rapidly in contused spinal cords (Sandler and Tator 1976; Dow-Edwards *et al.* 1982; Wallace and Tator 1986*a*). High-energy metabolites at the lesion site also fall, consistent with ischaemia (Anderson *et al.* 1976, 1980*a*,*b*, 1982; Braughler and Hall 1983*a*; Walker *et al.* 1977, 1979). Blood-flow in the white matter, however, is delayed by several hours (Senter and Venes 1978, 1979; Cawthon *et al.* 1980; Young *et al.* 1981, 1982*a*, *b*, *c*, 1986; Young and Flamm 1982). The post-traumatic fall in white matter blood-flow depends on injury severity. Moderate contusions of the spinal cord, for example, may elevate white matter blood-flow (Kobrine 1976; Lohse *et al.* 1980). Since autoregulation is disabled at the injury site (Young *et al.* 1982), systemic pressure changes (Young *et al.* 1980) may influence post-traumatic spinal blood-flow (Wallace and Tator 1987).

Neurophysiological monitoring of ascending and descending evoked responses in contused spinal cords showed a temporal pattern that correlated with the timing of blood-flow changes (Young *et al.* 1980). Contusion immediately abolishes somatosensory evoked potentials and descending vestibular responses conducting across the impact site. This even occurs with contusions that are not sufficient to produce lasting neurological deficits in the animals. However, with moderate trauma created by a 20 gm weight dropped 20 cm on to unsupported thoracic spinal cords, evoked potentials began recovering at 1–2 hours, only to fade again and permanently between 2 and 3 hours after injury. Recent studies suggest that the initial loss of evoked potentials is related to K released by traumatized cells (Young *et al.* 1982*b*). Extracellular K activity ($[K^+]_e$) rises from normal levels of 3–4 mM to >54 mM shortly after injury. $[K^+]_e$ recovers to normal in white matter at the lesion by 1–2 hours, at which time some evoked responses begin conducting across the injury. At 2–3 hours, when white matter blood flow falls to <6 ml/100gm/minute, the evoked responses disappear again.

A cause–effect relationship between blood-flow and spinal injury outcome, however, has not been firmly established. While the degree of post-traumatic white matter hypoperfusion increases with greater injury severity (Cawthon *et al.* 1980), it is not clear that the fall in blood-flow causes further tissue damage. Since substantial primary tissue damage occurs at the injury site, the fall in blood-flow may reflect rather than cause secondary injury. In addition, metabolic derangements occur rapidly at the injury site (Anderson *et al.* 1976, 1980*b*, 1982), preceding the fall in white matter blood-flow. Finally, white matter blood-flow falls only by 50–60 per cent by 3 hours after injury. Spinal cord white matter normally can tolerate flow losses of this magnitude without permanent damage. Thus, it is important to keep in mind that correlation does not necessarily imply causation.

Experimental treatments of acute spinal cord injury

The recognition that progressive tissue damage occurs in injured spinal cords provided the first rationale for acute spinal injury treatments. Many different treatments have been tried over the past three decades, ranging from hypothermia (Albin *et al.* 1968, 1969) and electromagnetic fields (Borgens *et al.* 1986*a*, *b*, 1987; Wallace *et al.* 1987*a*, *c*) to drugs (cf. Young 1985*a*) given shortly after injury. In addition, many models of spinal cord injury have been used, including the standard Allen weight drop contusion, compression (Anderson *et al.* 1976, 1980*a*, *b*, 1982, 1985), crush (Tator *et al.* 1984; Guha *et al.* 1985, 1987*a*, *b*; Wallace *et al.* 1986*a*, *b*, 1987*a*, *b*, *c*), and even ischaemia produced by occlusion of the descending thoracic aorta (Faden *et al.* 1983*a*, *c*; Faden and Jacobs 1985). Many different outcome measures have been used as criteria for therapeutic efficacy, ranging from blood-flow and biochemical measurements to neurophysiological and locomotory recovery.

Several drugs have been reported to improve post-traumatic blood-flow in injured spinal cords. Initial studies focused on antifibrinolytic (Campbell *et al.* 1974) and vasodilatory (Dow-Edwards *et al.* 1980) agents. By 1987 several other classes of drugs were found to prevent the post-traumatic fall in blood-flow. These include high doses of naloxone (Young *et al.* 1981; Faden *et al.* 1981), methylprednisolone (Anderson *et al.* 1982; Young *et al.* 1981), thyrotropin releasing hormone or TRH (Faden *et al.* 1981*a*, *b*, 1983), kappa opiate receptor blockers (Faden 1984; Faden and Jacobs 1985), Ca channel blockers (Guha *et al.* 1985, 1987), 21-aminosteroids (Hall *et al.* 1988), and others (Hall and Wolf 1986). Figure 2.1 summarizes the results of several studies from our laboratory on the effects of different drugs on spinal white matter blood-flow at 3 hours after contusion injury (Young *et al.* 1981; Young and Flamm 1982; Dow-Edwards *et al.* 1982). Normally, white matter spinal blood-flow is 12–14 ml/100 gm/minute, measured by hydrogen clearance in cats (Young 1980). At 3 hours after a 20 gm–20 cm weight drop contusion, it falls to 5–6 ml/100 gm/minute. Naloxone (10 mg/kg), methylprednisolone (15 mg/kg, 30 mg/kg), and aminophyllin and isoproterenol significantly improved white matter blood-flow.

Some of the drugs which prevented the delayed fall in spinal white matter blood-flow after injury also improved functional recovery. The first of these to be reported were naloxone (Faden *et al.* 1980; Flamm *et al.* 1982; Faden *et al.* 1982; Arias 1987) and methylprednisolone (Campbell *et al.* 1974;

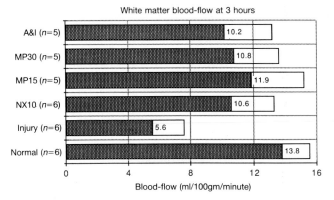

Fig. 2.1. White matter blood-flow measured at 3 hours after a 20 gm–20 cm contusion injury in untreated cats (Injury); after 10 mg/kg of naloxone (NX10, Young *et al.* 1981); 15 mg/kg and 30 mg/kg of methylprednisolone (MP15, MP30; Young and Flamm 1982); and aminophyllin and isoproterenol (A & I, Dow-Edwards *et al.* 1982). These are compared with white matter blood-flow in uninjured (Normal) animals. At 3 hours after a 20 gm–20 cm contusion, white matter blood-flow measured at the lesion site falls to <50 per cent of normal. NX10, MP15, MP30, and A & I all significantly improved this flow.

Young *et al.* 1988). Several related substances have also been reported to be beneficial, including TRH (Faden *et al.* 1981) and kappa opiate receptor blockers (Faden *et al.* 1984). Figure 2.2 summarizes the results of our studies on naloxone and methylprednisolone given 45 minutes after a 20 gm–20 cm weight drop contusion of the thoracic spinal cord (Young 1987; Flamm *et al.* 1986). In doses of 1 mg/kg and 3 mg/kg naloxone did not significantly improve recovery of locomotion. In doses of 10 mg/kg naloxone reduced the proportion of paralysed animals from a control level of 83 per cent in untreated animals to 35 per cent. Methylprednisolone (15 mg/kg) also appeared effective, reducing the proportion of paralysed animals to 22 per cent, as shown in Fig. 2.3. Somatosensory evoked potentials likewise showed a similar trend, as shown in Fig. 2.4. Incidentally, combined high dose naloxone (10 mg/kg) and methylprednisolone (15 mg/kg) significantly increased mortality in spinal-injured cats (Young *et al.* 1988).

As more laboratories gained experience with these drugs, however, it became clear that the treatment effects are not robust as initially thought. Some laboratories found no significant effects of high doses of naloxone (Wallace and Tator 1986*a*, *b*; Haghighi and Chehrazi 1987) or cortico-steroids (Faden *et al.* 1984) on their injury models. Drug effects differed depending on the injury model. For example, naloxone but not TRH improved functional recovery in a model of spinal cord ischaemia (Faden *et al.* 1982, 1983; Long *et al.* 1986). Discrepancies in therapeutic results have

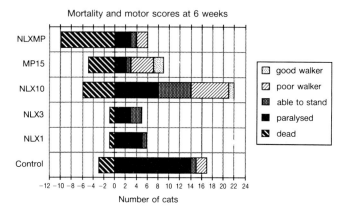

Fig. 2.2. Summary of locomotory recovery of cats at 6 weeks after a 20 gm weight drop 20 cm on to unsupported T8 spinal cord exposed by laminectomy. The number of animals that are walking well, walking poorly, only standing, paralysed, or dead are indicated for each treatment group. The Control group received saline, the NLX1, NLX3, and NLX10 groups respectively received 1 mg/kg, 3 mg/kg, and 10 mg of naloxone intravenously at 45 minutes and 3 hours after injury. The MP15 group received 15 mg/kg of methylprednisolone sodium succinate at 45 minutes and 3 hours after injury. The NLXMP group received 10 mg/kg of naloxone and 15 mg/kg of methylprednisolone (Figure adapted from Young *et al.* 1988).

been attributed to differences in anesthaesia, methods of evaluating functional and morphological outcome, and drug regimens tested. In many cases, data are simply not available. The only two drugs that have been studied by more than one laboratory are naloxone and methylprednisolone. Even the staunchest advocate of acute spinal cord injury treatments today would agree that treatment effects depend greatly on injury conditions, drug dosage and timing.

The first national acute spinal cord injury study

Laboratory studies of acute spinal cord injury treatments have reached an impasse. The proof of the pudding requires the demonstration that these drugs improve functional recovery in human spinal cord injury. Given the uncertainty of applying animal spinal cord injury results to the human condition, a clinical study is essential. In 1984, at the time that this situation was realized, a double-masked randomized clinical trial was already under way, comparing two doses of methylprednisolone (1 gm vs. 0.1 gm given intravenously daily, starting within 48 hours after injury and continued for 10 days). This study, called the National Acute Spinal Cord Injury Study I (NASCIS I), involved more than 300 patients at 10 centres. The patients were followed with neurological examinations for up to a year after injury.

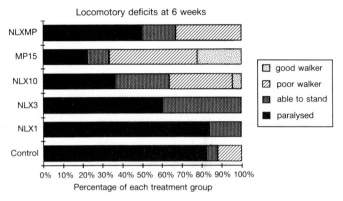

Fig. 2.3. Locomotory deficits of cats at 6 weeks after injury with 20 gm–20 cm weight drop contusion of the T8 spinal cord. Less than 20 per cent of the untreated (Control) cats recovered ability to walk or stand. Low doses of naloxone (1 mg/kg, NLX1) were not different from controls. Although nearly 40 per cent of cats treated with 3 mg/kg (NLX3) recovered ability to stand, none walked, and the differences were not stastically different from control ($p>0.05$, Chi square). More than 60 per cent of the 10 mg/kg naloxone treated cats (NLX10) recovered either standing or walking, with >50 per cent being able to walk; this is significantly different from control ($p<0.05$, Chi square). This conclusion holds even if we assume that all the animals that died before the sixth week would not have recovered any function. Methyprednisolone at 15 mg/kg (MP15) significantly improved the proportion of recovering animals. If we assume that all the animals that died would not have recovered, the results are less significant than the NLX10 results, but still significant ($p<0.05$, Chi square).

NASCIS I (Bracken *et al.* 1984, 1985) indicated no statistically significant differences between the neurological outcomes of spinal-injured patients treated with 1000 mg and 100 mg of methylprednisolone given within 48 hours after injury and then daily for 10 days. Figure 2.5 shows the time course of motor recovery in the patients, expressed in terms of their summed motor scores. Note the trend for improvement of motor scores in both groups. In general, all the patients improved significantly after spinal cord injury. Although patients treated with the higher dose of methylprednisolone tended to have better scores than the lower-dose group, the differences were not statistically significant, as shown in Fig. 2.6, which summarizes the sensory and motor examination results at one year after injury, showing the changes in motor and sensory scores between admission and the one-year follow-up examination.

The NASCIS I trial has been criticized in four respects. First, the drug may have been given too late. Most laboratory studies, with one exception (Faden *et al.* 1982*b*), tested earlier (<1 hour after injury) treatments. Almost no patient in the study received drug within an hour, the majority were treated more than 3 hours after injury, and some were treated for as long as 24–48 hours after

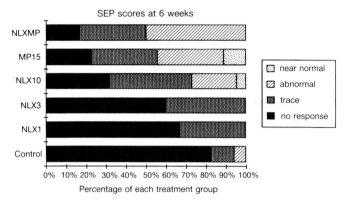

Fig. 2.4. Somatosensory evoked potentials in cats at 6 weeks after a 20 gm–20 cm weight drop contusion of the spinal cord. Less than 20 per cent of the untreated injured group (Control) recovered responses, while there was a trend for fewer animals with no responses, i.e. 68 per cent, 60 per cent, and 32 per cent in animals treated with 1 mg/kg (NLX1), 3 mg/kg (NLX3), and 10 mg/kg (NLX10) of naloxone. The animals treated with 15 mg/kg of methylprednisolone (MP15) had the lowest percentage of non-responders, at 24 per cent, but this result is not as impressive if we assume that all the animals that died before 6 weeks did not recover (Figure adapted from Young *et al.* 1988).

injury. Second, the doses were variable, and possibly insufficient. The patients received 1000 or 100 mg of doses regardless of body weight. Depending on body weight, a patient in the high-dose group thus may have received 10–15 mg/kg. Laboratory experiments suggest that the optimal dose in about 30 mg/kg (Braughler and Hall 1985). Third, different spinal cord injuries were lumped together, ranging from complete cervical spinal cord injury to incomplete lumbo-sacral injuries. The responses of such a diverse population to treatment are likely to be quite different. Finally, the trial compared high- and low-dose treatments. It does not address the question whether the treatment outcome is significantly different compared to placebo. Given the lateness of the treatments, the variability of the doses, and the variety of spinal cord injuries that are lumped together, a negative result is not too surprising.

The second national acute spinal cord injury study

In 1984, the two most promising treatments from animal studies were high doses of methylprednisolone (Demopoulos *et al.* 1981; Hall *et al.* 1984) and naloxone (Faden *et al.* 1980; Young *et al.* 1981). After phase I clinical trials showing that 5.4 mg/kg doses of naloxone (Flamm *et al.* 1985) and 30 mg/kg doses of methylprednisolone (Young *et al.* 1988) were safe in spinal-injured

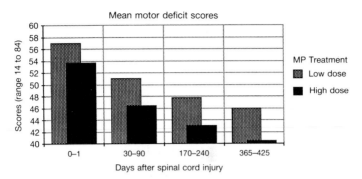

Fig. 2.5. Motor deficits in humans (adapted from Bracken *et al.* 1984) at different times after injury, comparing 150 patients treated with high-dose (1 gm given within 48 hours after injury and 1 gm daily for 10 days) and low-dose (100 mg given within 48 hours after injury and 100 mg daily for 10 days) methylprednisolone. Note the trend for improvement in both groups. Although the high-dose group had less motor deficit from the low-dose group, the difference between the two groups was not statistically significant (Figure adapted from Bracken *et al.* 1986).

humans, the second national acute spinal cord injury study (NASCIS II) was initiated in 1985 to test three predictions: (1) that methylprednisolone or naloxone will significantly improve recovery compared to placebo; (2) that earlier treatment is more effective than late; and (3) that treatment is less effective in patients with no versus partial motor or sensory preservation.

At 10 centres, 487 patients were randomized to three treatment arms:

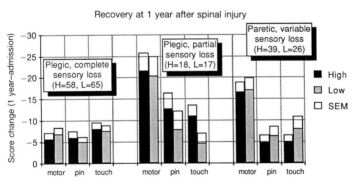

Fig. 2.6. Recovery of sensory and motor responses in humans at 1 year after injury (adapted from Bracken *et al.* 1986), comparing 115 patients treated with high-dose (1 gm within 48 hours after injury and 1 gm daily for 10 days) and 108 patients treated with low-dose (100 mg within 48 hours and 100 mg daily for 10 days) methyl-prednisolone. There was no significant difference in the motor deficit scores, pinprick, and touch-sensory scores of the two groups (Figure adapted from Bracken *et al.* 1986).

methylprednisolone (30 mg/kg bolus followed by a 5.4 mg/kg/hour for 23 hours), naloxone (5.4 mg/kg bolus followed by 4.0 mg/kg/hour for 23 hours), and placebo (vehicles for the two drugs). Mean admission and treatment times were 3.1 and 8.7 hours after injury, with 92 per cent receiving drug according to protocol. On admission, 6 weeks, 6 months, and 1 year after injury, 14 muscle groups were graded on a scale of 0 to 5 for a total of 0 to 70 motor points on each side of the body. Dermatomes were graded for pin and touch sensation on a scale of 0 to 2 indicating no, abnormal, or normal sensation. Admission neurological scores were very similar in the three groups. However, the methylprednisolone group had more 'complete' patients than the naloxone or placebo groups, 64 per cent, 53 per cent, and 58 per cent respectively. Although not statistically significant, this difference would reduce neurological recovery in the methylprednisolone group.

NASCIS II (Bracken *et al.* 1990) showed that methylprednisolone-treated patients recovered more motor and sensory function than placebo-treated patients at 6 weeks, 6 months, and one year after injury. Neither drug significantly increased mortality or morbidity. Naloxone-treated patients did not differ significantly from placebo-treated patients. Three further analyses were done. First, patients treated within 8 hours were compared with those treated more than 8 hours after injury. Neither drug was effective when given more than 8 hours after injury. Second, patients treated within 8 hours were segregated into those with complete neurological loss (plegic) and those with some sensory or motor preservation (paretic). At 6 weeks after injury, placebo-treated plegic patients lost an average of 54.4 motor points and recovered 1.3 points, i.e. a 2 per cent recovery. Methylprednisolone-treated plegic patients lost 53.1 motor points and recovered 12 per cent, significantly more than placebo ($p<0.021$). Paretic placebo-treated patients lost 21.8 motor points and recovered 50 per cent compared to 56 per cent—not statistically significant ($p<0.054$). At 6 months, placebo-treated plegic patients recovered 8 per cent compared to 20 per cent in methylprednisolone-treated patients ($p<0.020$) while paretic placebo-treated patients recovered 59 per cent compared to 75 per cent ($p<0.018$). Comparing only protocol-compliant patients, the differences were still significant, i.e. motor ($p<0.011$), pin ($p<0.001$), and touch ($p<0.020$).

High-dose methylprednisolone therefore improved motor and sensory recovery when given within 8 hours after injury. It was not beneficial when given more than 8 hours after injury. It improved recovery in both 'plegic' and 'paretic' patients. Thus, the results support our first two hypotheses that methylprednisolone can improve recovery and that earlier treatment is better. The finding that treatment improved recovery in both 'plegic' and 'paretic' patients was not anticipated.

NASCIS II is the first demonstration that any drug improves recovery in human spinal cord injury. Secondary injury has long been suspected from animal spinal cord injury studies; but the NASCIS results strongly suggest that it occurs in humans as well. It appears not only that we can reduce secondary injury, but that we have less than eight hours to do so. The eight hours is based on the median treatment time in the study. The treatment-time window is probably shorter than eight hours, and may apply not only to drugs but to surgical therapy of acute spinal cord injury as well. Finally, both 'plegic' and 'paretic' patients benefited from the treatment, suggesting that 'complete' injury is *not* complete.

Methylprednisolone is not an ideal drug for spinal cord injury. The treatment effects were modest. In the NASCIS II protocol, as much as 10 g of methylprednisolone was administered to patients over 24 hours, a massive dose by any standard. While NASCIS II detected no deleterious side-effects, such large doses of a potent corticosteroid drug are unlikely to be entirely innocuous, and some side-effect may emerge with larger numbers of patients. The search for a more potent and specific drug has begun. One new drug looks promising: tirilazad mesylate (McCall *et al.* 1987). This 21-aminosteroid is approximately 100 times more potent than methylprednisolone as a lipid peroxidation inhibitor and has no corticosteriod receptor activity (Hall *et al.* 1989). Animal studies suggest therapeutic benefit of this drug in spinal cord injury (Anderson *et al*, 1988; Braughler and Hall 1989; Hall and Braughler 1989; Hall *et al.* 1989).

The finding of an effective therapy has complicated further trials. If methylprednisolone significantly improves neurological recovery in patients, future clinical trials cannot ethically use placebo controls. Clinical trials must compare against methylprednisolone and animal studies must demonstrate that a new treatment is equal to or better than methylprednisolone before it can be considered for clinical trial. Since differences between two treatments will be smaller than between a treatment and placebo, investigators must study larger numbers of subjects or have more reliable outcome measures. Finally, combination or sequential treatments should be considered.

Opiate receptor mechanisms in neural injury

The mechanisms by which naloxone affects blood-flow and neurological outcome in spinal cord injury are not well understood. In their initial report Faden *et al.* (1980) attributed the beneficial effects of naloxone in spinal cord injury to improvements in systemic pressure. A subsequent study (Young *et al.* 1981) discounted this explanation, finding that the changes of blood-pressure were insufficient to explain the improvement of blood-flow by naloxone. Wallace and Tator (1986*a*, *b*) recently reopened the issue by reporting that naloxone did not improve cardiac output, spinal cord blood-flow, and neurological outcome (Wallace *et al.* 1986) after experimental spinal injury in rats. They did, however, find (Wallace and Tator 1987) that raising blood-pressure and cardiac output can improve spinal blood-flow.

The effect of naloxone on spinal cord injury was found serendipitously.

Although the beneficial effects of high-dose naloxone on functional recovery in spinal cord injury continues to be debated, the findings have greatly stimulated the field. Partly as a consequence, more spinal cord injury studies have been done in the past decade than in all preceding years. For example, owing to the interest in establishing treatment effects, the first quantitative studies of biochemical, morphological, neurophysiological, and behavioural outcomes of spinal cord injury were carried out. The discovery that naloxone may have a beneficial effect on spinal cord injury opened a door to the possibility that opiate receptors play a role in other types of neural injury. Shortly after the first reports that naloxone may be beneficial in spinal cord injury, Hosobuchi *et al.* (1982) suggested its use in stroke. Although the evidence supporting this suggestion in cerebral ischaemia is quite controversial (Kastin *et al.* 1982; Holaday and D'Amato 1982), positive results of naloxone treatment of several ischaemia models have been reported (Turner *et al.* 1984; Faden *et al.* 1983).

The doses of naloxone required to have an effect on injured spinal cords are in the range of 2–10 mg/kg, 100–1000 times greater than that necessary to block opiate receptors. For example, a 0.5 mg total dose (<0.008 mg/kg for a typical 70 kg person) of naloxone will effectively reverse heroin overdose in a patient. Naloxone may be acting through mechanisms unrelated to its normally accepted action as a specific blocker of μ opiate receptors. To explain the high doses of naloxone necessary to reduce the neural injury Faden *et al.* (1985) proposed that the effects of naloxone in neural injury are related to blockade of the kappa opiate receptor. Since naloxone does not bind kappa receptors as avidly as it does mu receptors, very large doses are required. Faden *et al.* (1983*a*, *b*) reported that the more specific kappa antagonists such as TRH and WIN44,441–3 also have beneficial effects on spinal ischaemia models. These findings have not yet been confirmed by other laboratories.

Regardless of the type of opiate receptor that naloxone and TRH are acting on, the question of how blockade of opiate receptors protects traumatized spinal cords remains unanswered. The site of action of naloxone and TRH in spinal cord injury has yet to be defined. The possibility that it may be indirect, perhaps through systemic pressure changes or release of some intermediate substance, has not been ruled out. The role of opiate receptor blockers in the treatment of endotoxic shock or haemorrhagic shock, however, is rapidly gaining wide acceptance (Holaday and Faden 1978; Faden and Holaday 1979; Holaday and Faden 1980). Trauma causes the release of many systemic substances, including glucocorticosteroids, endogenous opioids, catecholamines, serotonin, monokines, lymphokines, and stress-related proteins. High doses of opiate receptor blockers influence the synthesis and release of these substances both peripherally and centrally. These substances may modulate the spinal cord response to injury in ways that we do not yet understand.

Lipid peroxidation: an autodestructive mechanism

Methylprednisolone played a crucial role in stimulating the current interest in lipid peroxidation mechanisms in spinal cord injury. Although the concept of using high-dose methylprednisolone treatment as an antioxidant to scavenge free radicals has been extant some years (Campbell *et al.* 1974; Demopoulos *et al.* 1980, 1981), recent studies opened up other possibilities. High doses of methylprednisolone (15–30 mg/kg) inhibit lipid peroxidation (Braughler and Hall 1981*a, b*; Hall and Braughler, 1981, 1982; Anderson *et al.* 1985; Braughler and Hall 1985), reduce metabolic derangements (Braughler and Hall 1983*a*), protect ATPase activity (Braughler and Hall 1981*a, b*, 1984) and prevent neurofilament loss in injured spinal cords (Braughler and Hall 1984). In addition, corticosteroids may directly or indirectly inhibit phospholipase A_2 activity (Metz *et al.* 1980; Hirata *et al.* 1980). While the optimal dose for reducing lipid peroxidation is 30 mg/kg, doubling the dose to 60 mg/kg not only is less effective but may aggravate lipid peroxidation. The effect of methylprednisolone on blood-flow (Braughler and Hall 1981*b*, 1982, 1983*b*; Hall and Braughler 1982; Hall *et al.* 1983, 1984; Braughler *et al.* 1987) and Gram-negative bacterial sepsis (Greisman 1982) had similar dose–response curves.

Braughler and Hall (1985) proposed that the therapeutic effects of methylprednisolone on spinal cord injury stemmed not from its glucocorticosteroid activity but rather its chemical ability to inhibit lipid peroxidation. This would explain why such large doses are necessary and why the drug has such a narrow dose–response curve. This proposal provided the rationale for the development of a new family of potent lipid peroxidation inhibitor drugs called 21-aminosteroids (Hall *et al.* 1987). These drugs have no glucocorticosteroid activity, but are more potent inhibitors of lipid peroxidation than methylprednisolone. Studies are now being carried out with 21-aminosteroid drugs in spinal cord injury models.

Of the many proposed mechanisms of secondary injury lipid peroxidation has attracted the most attention, because it promises to tie together many potential causes of tissue damage and ischaemia in one unifying sequence of events. Injury causes Ca ions to rush into cells, disrupting mitochondrial electron transport (Chance 1965) and activating phospholipases (Braughler *et al.* 1985*a*; Young 1985*b*). Injured mitochondria generate oxygen free radicals which attack membrane and enhance phospholipase-mediated breakdown of membranes, releasing lipid peroxides and free arachidonic acid (Braughler *et al.* 1985*b*). Free arachidonic acid is enzymatically converted to prostaglandins and leukotrienes, some of which are among the most potent vasoactive substances known in biology (Kontos *et al.* 1981; Pickard 1981; Wolfe 1982; Feuerstein *et al.* 1987) and can cause pathological and biochemical changes similar to those observed in traumatized or ischaemic tissues (Chan and Fishman 1980*a, b*, 1985; Chan *et al.* 1983,

1984). Several laboratories have found elevated levels of vasoconstrictive prostaglandins and lipid peroxides in injured spinal cords (Hsu *et al.* 1985; Horrocks *et al.* 1985; Saunders *et al.* 1987). Thus, treatments that prevent lipid peroxidation may be able to affect secondary injury processes on several levels.

The eicosanoids may mediate much of the spinal cord injury response to trauma. For example, prostacyclin (PGI_2), a primary cycloxygenase metabolite of arachidonic acid in endothelial cells, is a very potent inhibitor of platelet aggregation, and one of the most powerful vasodilating agents known (Kontos *et al.* 1981). PGI_2 is released rapidly by injured endothelial cells, possibly causing the early hyperaemia that is often observed in spinal cord injury (McIntire *et al.* 1985). Its release is modulated by many factors (Feuerstein *et al.* 1987), i.e. thrombin, bradykinin, histamine, ephinephrine, angiotensin II, ATP/ADP ratios, acetylcholine, oxygen radicals, serotonin, endotoxin, monokines (Rossi *et al.* 1985), lymphokines (interleukin-2), and Ca ions. Thromboxane A_2 (TXA_2), a platelet-derived product of arachidonic acid metabolism, is also released by endothelial cells, but at a slower rate than PGI_2. TXA_2 opposes PGI_2 activities, promoting platelet aggregation, thrombosis, and vasoconstriction. It may mediate the delayed fall in white matter blood-flow. Other products of arachidonic acid metabolism include the leukotrienes, generated by 5-lipoxygenase. Produced by neutrophils, some leukotrienes, particularly LTC_4/D_4 and LTB_4, increase postcapillary venule permeability and can contribute to oedema. Several recent studies of injured spinal cords have shown marked increases in TXA_2 and LTC_4/D_4 and B_4, as well as a decrease in PGI_2 at the injury site (Demediuk *et al.* 1985; Saunders *et al.* 1987). Drugs are available for manipulating the enzymes responsible for eicosanoid production as well as the eicosanoid receptors.

Ca ions: a final common pathway of cell death?

Normally, intracellular Ca ionic activity ($[Ca^{+2}]_i$) is extremely low, <0.1 μM, while extracellular Ca ionic activity ($[Ca^{+2}]_e$) is usually >1.0 mM. Because of this enormous gradient, Ca ions rush into injured neurons. Since Ca ions regulate many biological processes, including cellular transport, secretion and synaptic transmission, mitosis, and cell growth, excessive Ca entry should be thoroughly disruptive, if not fatal to cells. In addition, elevated $[Ca^{+2}]_i$ activate phospholipases which in turn break down membrane and release free arachidonic acid for prostaglandin production, shunt mitochondrial electrons to oxygen and other free radicals (Braughler *et al.* 1985*a, b*), and ultimately interfere with all phosphorylation reactions. Some investigators have called Ca entry into cells the final common pathway of cell death (Schanne *et al.* 1979).

Much evidence supports a central role of Ca ions in the response of spinal cords to injury (Young 1986). $[Ca^{+2}]_e$ falls to very low levels shortly after injury, to <0.01 mM, and remains depressed <0.1 mM for many hours in injured spinal cords (Young *et al.* 1982*a*; Young and Flamm 1982*b*). Using atomic absorption spectroscopy, we (Young and Koreh 1986) and others (Balentine and Spector 1977; Happel *et al.* 1981; Happel *et al.* 1984) have found large increases in total tissue Ca concentrations, $[Ca]_t$, at the lesion site. Within 3 hours after a contusion injury, $[Ca]_t$ increases as much as 50 per cent, as shown in Fig. 2.7. Combined, these findings indicate that large amounts of Ca are being bound and precipitate at the injury site. Superfusion of spinal cords with hypercalcic solutions or Ca iontophores produces pathological lesions in spinal cord similar to those caused by trauma or ischaemia (Balentine and Dean 1982; Balentine 1983). Finally, both electron- and light-microscopic studies indicate the presence of Ca deposits in injured axons at the lesion site of traumatized spinal cords (Balentine and Hilton 1980; Balentine and Green 1984). Given the ability of Ca influx to initiate lipid peroxidation and stimulate pathological prostaglandins production, it is likely that the initial Ca influx into cells is a trigger for the cascade of necrotic events that occur after spinal cord injury.

The magnitudes of the $[Ca^{+2}]_e$ fall Ca accumulation at the lesion site are much than expected. Figure 2.8 shows a summary of $[Ca^{+2}]_e$ changes at and around the injury site of a injured spinal cord (Young *et al.* 1980*b*). At the lesion centre, $[Ca^{+2}]_e$ falls precipitously to as low as 0.001 mM within seconds after a 20 gm–20 cm weight drop impact, recovering slowly to about 0.01 mM by 4 hours. In white matter at the lesion centre, $[Ca^{+2}]_e$ also falls to very low levels, to <0.01 mM, but recovers transiently to about 0.4 mM and falls to <0.1 mM by 3 hours. A simple calculation indicates that this fall of $[Ca^{+2}]_e$ cannot be due to equilibration of Ca ions between the

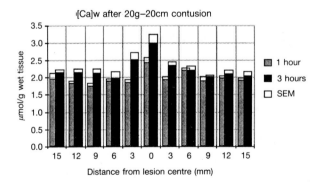

Fig. 2.7. Distribution of mean total tissue Ca concentrations ([Ca]w) in two groups of 8 cats, studied at 1 and 3 hours after 20 gm–20 cm contusion of the thoracic spinal cord. The spinal cords were cut into 3 mm segments, centred on the lesion site. At 1 hour, there was a significant increase in [Ca]w at the lesion centre (0 mm). Normal [Ca]w is about 2.1 μmol/gm wet tissue weight (Figure adapted from Young and Koreh 1986).

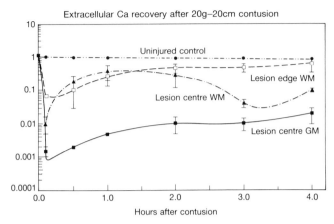

Fig. 2.8. Mean extracellular Ca ionic activity ($[Ca^{+2}]_e$) in 9 cats. Normally (Uninjured control, $n = 3$), $[Ca^{+2}]_e$ is 1.0–1.2 mM, and does not change over a three-hour period after laminectomy. In grey matter at the lesion centre (Lesion centre GM), $[Ca^{+2}]_e$ fell rapidly to nearly 1 μmol, and recovered slowly to about 10 μmol. In white matter adjacent at the lesion centre (Lesion centre (GM), $[Ca^{+2}]_e$ fell to 10 mM, recovered to 0.4 mM, and then fell again to <0.1 mM at 2–3 hours. In white matter at the lesion edge (Lesion edge WM) 10 mm from the lesion centre, $[Ca^{+2}]_e$ also fell to <0.1 mM, but recovered rapidly and steadily (Figure adapted from Young *et al.* 1982*c*).

intra- and extracellular space alone. Assuming that $[Ca^{+2}]_i$ is essentially 0 mM, $[Ca^{+2}]_e$ is 1.2 mM, and the extracellular volume fraction is about 15 per cent before injury, complete mixing of the intra- and extracellular compartments should result in a fall of $[Ca^{+2}]_e$ to about 0.2 mM, not 1–10 μM. Likewise, if $[Ca^{+2}]_e$ is normally 1.2 mM and the extracellular volume fraction is 15 per cent, there should only be 0.18 μmol of extracellular Ca ions per gm of tissue. Since total Ca concentration increases by as much as 1.0 μmol/gm by 3 hours after injury, we can conclude that the Ca accumulated represent more than five times the amount of Ca originally present at the lesion site.

Ca ions are probably entering injured cells through many routes besides Ca channels. From a therapeutic point of view, Ca entry into injured axons in the spinal cord will be difficult to control with Ca channel blockers. Furthermore, since Ca ions are universal intracellular messengers for many biological processes, any drug which effectively blocks Ca entry into cells is likely to have many profound and confounding side-effects on the peripheral system before any major central effect occurs. At higher doses sufficient to block neuronal Ca channels, however, Ca channel blockers ultimately should be imcompatible with life. However, Ca channel blockers may have some beneficial effects at low doses. For example, Ca channel blockers can dilate blood-vessels, and may improve blood-flow at the lesion site (Guha *et al.* 1985, 1987).

Protective mechanisms against excessive Ca entry

The concept of secondary injury mechanisms, and particularly the role of Ca, presents us with a perplexing question. Why have organisms evolved elaborate autodestructive mechanisms that are inimical to their survival? Neurons are the most critical and longest-living cells of the body. Yet they are exquisitely Ca-sensitive, and live in a sea of Ca ions waiting to rush in and trigger destruction at the slightest injury. Although this situation may have been an unwitting development due to the evolution of Ca ions as a universal intracellular messenger, organisms must have evolved effective mechanisms to protect their neurons against excessive Ca entry. Measurements of $[Ca^{+2}]_e$ and $[Ca]_t$ provide some insight into what these mechanisms may be in spinal cord injury.

$[Ca^{+2}]_e$ invariably falls in injured central nervous tissues, whether the injury is due to trauma or ischaemia. In spinal cord injury, $[Ca^{+2}]_e$ falls from normal levels of >1000 μM to <10 μM, remaining <100 μM for many hours after injury. $[Ca]_t$ rises twofold by 3 hours, and to as high as eight times normal values at 24 hours after injury. Some substance(s) must therefore be binding and precipitating large amounts of Ca. This substance must be available in sufficient concentration to bind 20–30 μmoles of Ca per gram of wet tissue. It must bind Ca strongly enough to buffer $[Ca^{+2}]_e$ to 1 μM. Furthermore, because $[Ca^{+2}]_e$ remains depressed for many hours, there must be continuing release of this substance for long periods of time, capable of precipitating the Ca ions diffusing to the lesion site from surrounding tissues and blood. Few substances meet these stringent criteria (Young 1987). While some proteins, i.e. calmodulin, bind Ca ions at concentrations of <0.1 μM, they are not present in mM concentrations. Other substances are present in sufficient concentration but do not bind such low concentrations of Ca, for example, amino acids.

One class of substances, however, meet these criteria: the phosphates. Central nervous tissues contain very high levels of phosphates. For example, in spinal cord, total tissue phosphate is 150–170 mM. About 20 mM are inorganic phosphates and labile organophosphates, such as ATP, ADP, and phosphocreatine. Most of the remainder, probably >70 per cent, reside in membrane phospholipids. Inorganic phosphates (PO_4) bind Ca, forming many possible intermediate Ca phosphate complexes, with hydroxyapatite being thermodynamically the most stable end-product (Matheja and Degens 1971; Brown 1971). Although inorganic phosphate species that bind Ca most avidly (e.g. PO_4^{-3} and polyphosphates) usually comprise a small fraction of the inorganic phosphate pool under normal conditions (Chughtai et al. 1968), precipitation with Ca will shift the equilibrium to generate more of these species. Also, by-products of phospholipid breakdown, i.e. phosphoethanolamine and phosphocholine) and lipid peroxides will bind Ca ions at <1 μM. Phospholipid breakdown in injured cells should release sufficient inorganic phosphates and by-products of phospholipid breakdown to buffer $[Ca^{+2}]_e$ to 1–10 µM (Young 1987).

Rapid lowering of $[Ca^{+2}]_e$ in ischaemic and traumatized nervous tissues should protect cells that survive the primary injury by reducing the gradient driving Ca ionic entry into cells. This mechanism possesses several attractive features. First, it is initiated by Ca entry into cells, activating phospholipases and free-radical breakdown of membrane phospholipids. Second, because of the high concentrations of phosphates in central nervous tissues, the rapid and complete autodestruction of a relatively small proportion of the cells will yield sufficient phosphates to buffer and maintain $[Ca^{+2}]_e$ at very low levels. Third, the mechanism is robust and does not require metabolic energy, which may be in short supply in injured tissues. Fourth, substrates for this mechanism are present in all cells. Finally, some by-products of phospholipid breakdown, e.g. prostaglandins and leukotrienes, cause vasoconstriction and cellular swelling. The latter reduces extracellular space through which Ca ions diffuse. Together, oedema and reduction of blood-flow will reduce the amount of Ca diffusing to the lesion site, and thereby help maintain $[Ca^{+2}]_e$ at low levels. Thus, by altruistically sacrificing some injured cells, central nervous tissues can enhance the survival of the remaining cells.

Calcium paradox: a mechanism of secondary injury

The profound and prolonged depression of $[Ca^{+2}]_e$ that occurs in injured spinal cords raises the possibility that 'Ca paradox' may be occurring in injured spinal cords. The Ca paradox phenomenon was first described in heart muscles. If an isolated heart is perfused with Ca-free solutions for a period of time and then restored to normal Ca-containing solutions, the heart will die (Zimmerman and Hulsmann 1966; Ruigrok *et al.* 1975; Hearse *et al.* 1978; Ashraf 1987; Kanaide *et al.* 1987). During the period of exposure to Ca-free solutions, cardiac cells become permeable to Ca, and Na ions will enter the cells (Alto and Dhalla 1979; Grinwald 1982; Hohl *et al.* 1983; Chapman *et al.* 1984; Ruano Arroyo *et al.* 1984; Busselen 1987). The critical $[Ca^{+2}]_e$ levels that produces this effect is about 10 µM for about 30 minutes (Baker *et al.* 1984; Oksendal *et al.* 1985; Hunt and Willis 1985). Upon restoration of normal $[Ca^{+2}]_e$ Ca ions rush into the cells, aided by exchange with Na ions accumulated in the cells during the low-Ca phase (Chapman *et al.* 1984; Nayler *et al.* 1984; Ruano Arroyo *et al.* 1984). Ca paradox causes pathological reactions in heart muscle that are reminiscent of spinal cord injury, including lipid peroxidation (Julicher *et al.* 1984), production of eicosanoids (Karmazyn 1987), and release of free radicals (Hearse *et al.* 1978; Hess and Manson 1984).

Although Ca paradox has yet to be demonstrated in neurons, all the essential elements of the reaction are present in the contused spinal cord (Young 1986). In contused spinal cords, $[Ca^{+2}]_e$ rapidly falls to <0.01 mM, not only at the impact site but as far as 1 cm away (Young *et al*. 1982*b*). At the impact centre, $[Ca^{+2}]_e$ remains depressed for many hours. However, in white matter at the lesion edge $[Ca^{+2}]_e$ recovers within 1–2 hours, only to fall again at 2–3 hours. Extracellular K activity rises to high levels (Young *et al*. 1982*a*). Na ions enter cells and accumulate at the lesion site (Young and DeCrescito 1986). Thus, the stage is set for a Ca paradox at the injury site. Rapid restoration of $[Ca^{+2}]_e$ may thus be paradoxically deleterious to injured spinal cords.

Treatments that have been found to protect the heart against Ca paradox bear strikingly similarities to treatments that have been reported to be beneficial in acute spinal cord injury. For example, hypothermia to 10°C increases the length of time that cardiac cells can be exposed to Ca-free solutions without showing Ca-paradox changes (Holland and Olsen 1975; Boink *et al*. 1980; Rich and Langer 1982; Baker *et al*. 1983; Baker and Hearse 1983*b*; Ganote and Sims 1984; Rudge and Duncan 1984). The Ca channel blockers, verapamil (Baker and Hearse, 1983*a*; Alanen *et al*. 1984; Eichelberg *et al*. 1984; Oksendal and Jynge 1986), diltiazem (Ashraf *et al*. 1982; Meno *et al*. 1984), ionic Ca blockers (Busselen 1985; Oksendal and Jynge 1986), and others (Baker and Hearse 1983*a*, 1985; Chapman *et al*. 1986; Koomen *et al*. 1983), reduce the damage produced by Ca paradox. Other treatments include adrenergic blockade (Oksendal and Jynge 1987; Hirata *et al*. 1984), reduction of extracellular Na (Busselen 1982, 1985, 1987), anaesthetic agents (Tunstall *et al*. 1986; Hoka *et al*. 1987), allopurinol (Oksendal *et al*. 1987), and chlorpromazine (Rabkin 1987).

The possibility that Ca paradox plays a role in secondary injury after spinal cord trauma carries several interesting therapeutic implications. First, restoration of blood-flow without concomitant measures to protect cells against further Ca entry may be deleterious. Second, since Ca paradox may take place over a period of hours after the initial trauma, this extends the time during which treatments may be effective. Third, a variety of therapeutic approaches have been reported to be beneficial for Ca paradox in the heart. Many of these have not yet been tried in the spinal cord. Finally, the existence of such a phenomenon may explain the narrow effective-dosage ranges that have been reported for methylprednisolone in spinal cord injury. At 10 mg/kg, methylprednisolone has relatively little effect on lipid peroxidation. The effect peaks at 30 mg/kg. At 60 mg/kg methylprednisolone has been reported to enhance lipid peroxidation injured spinal cords.

Conclusions

Central nervous tissues face a very difficult survival problem. Neurons are exquisitely sensitive to Ca ions, but live in a sea of Ca ions that threaten to invade with the slightest injury. Neurons also contain relatively high concentrations of K ions, and a variety of neurotransmitters. The former will depolarize neurons, opening voltage-sensitive Ca channels. The latter will activate receptor-related ionic channels through which Ca can pass. Traumatic injury disrupts cells, releasing K and neurotransmitters into the extracellular space. Elevated $[K^+]_e$ and neurotransmitters such as glutamate will depolarize and enhance Ca influx into neighbouring neurons. This extracellular environment must be deleterious to neurons that survive the trauma. Many of these neurons are probably partially injured and teetering on the borderline of survival, having shipped in sufficient Ca ions to depress their normal membrane pumping activity. Continued entry of Ca ions into these cells is likely to ensure their demise.

Central nervous tissues appeared to have evolved an elegant and effective mechanism to deal with this problem. By endowing cells with an abundance of Ca-activated phospholipases, the organism guarantees the rapid auto-destruction of injured cells, and complete release of their phosphates into extracellular space. As if this were not enough, Ca entry into cells will initiate supporting reactions which will hasten the complete destruction of the cells, including the release of free radicals and lysosomal protease enzymes that will dissolve membranes to expose any hidden phospholipids. It is perhaps no accident that spinal cord tissues contain very high concentrations of phosphates—170 mM, higher than almost any biological material except for egg yolk and some viral and bacterial particles. This provides more than sufficient phosphates to bind all the Ca ions in the extracellular space many times over. In fact, the complete release of phosphates from a small percentage of cells in the spinal cord should be more than sufficient to buffer $[Ca^{+2}]_e$ to 1 μM. This process has further advantages in that it does not require metabolic energy, intact membranes, or even living cells to proceed.

Lowering of $[Ca^{+2}]_e$ is unquestionably the most effective and efficient means of reducing Ca entry into surviving cells. Owing to the diversity of channels and other membrane openings by which Ca ions can enter cells, no subtance can effectively block Ca entry into partially injured cells. The safest route is to release a massive amount of a substance that can bind Ca ions and buffer $[Ca^{+2}]_e$ to very low levels, eliminating the steep ionic gradient that drives Ca ions into cells. This will provide a crucial margin of time during which injured neurons can repair breaks in their membrane, restore their metabolic supplies, and recoup their energies. The cells that are sacrificed in this process probably will not survive anyway. The tissue will also be rid of lingering moribund cells that would unnecessarily waste metabolic substrates and oxygen. This mechanism requires altruistic suicide of severely injured cells to improve the survival of less injured cells.

All the sacrifice of cells and phosphate release would be for naught if Ca ions were to pour into the lesion site from adjacent spinal cord and blood. When $[Ca^{+2}]_e$ at the lesion centre falls to <0.01 mM a large Ca ionic gradient develops between the lesion site and surrounding tissues. Is there a method for reducing the Ca diffusion to the lesion site? The only way in which this can be practically achieved is to restrict blood-flow and decrease the extracellular space through which Ca ions must diffuse. This, we suggest, is the function of the prostaglandins and leukotrienes generated from products of lipid breakdown. Some of these are among the most potent vasoactive and potent oedema-causing agents known in biology. Thromboxane A_2, for example, causes vasoconstriction and cellular swelling. The effectiveness of these agents is perhaps best illustrated by the prolonged depression of $[Ca^{+2}]_e$ at <0.1 mM at the lesion site, despite restoration of $[Ca^{+2}]_e$ to >1 mM in surrounding spinal cord.

In the end, however, even the best laid plans can backfire. The mechanism proposed above probably works best for moderate trauma injuries of the spinal cord. In severe injuries, where a large proportion of the cells at the lesion site are disrupted by trauma, the release of free radicals and prostaglandins may become excessive. The resultant oedema and vasoconstriction may cause further damage to surviving cells. This is probably the situation where drugs such as methylprednisolone have the most beneficial effects. On the other hand, complete suppression of lipid peroxidation and other components of this mechanism by which nervous tissues reduce $[Ca^{+2}]_e$ may lead to over-rapid restoration of $[Ca^{+2}]_e$ to the tissue, and Ca paradox reactions may result. This would explain the very narrow therapeutic range of most drugs that have been reported to be beneficial in spinal cord injury. Thus, therapy of acute spinal cord injury is unlikely to come in the form of a magic bullet that will be good for all injuries and under all circumstances. The object of therapy should be to achieve a balance between several conflicting mechanisms.

References

Alanen, K. A., Lipasti, J. A., Tasanne, M. R., and Nevalainen, T. J. (1984). Effect of verapamil on reperfusion damage and calcium paradox in isolated rat heart. *Experimental Pathology*, **25**(3), 131–8.

Albin, M. S., White, R. J., Acosta-Rua, G., and Yahon, D. (1968). Study of functional recovery produced by delayed localized cooling after spinal cord injury in primates. *Journal of Neurosurgery*, **29**, 113–20.

Albin, M. S., White, R. J., Yashon, D., and Harris, L. S. (1969). Effects of localized cooling on spinal cord trauma. *Journal of Trauma*, **9**, 1000–8.

Allen, A. R. (1911). Surgery of experimental lesion of spinal cord equivalent to crush injury of fracture dislocation. *Journal of the American Medical Association*, **50**, 941–52.

Allen, A. R. (1914). Remarks on histopathological changes in spinal cord due to impact: an experimental study. *Journal of Nervous and Mental Diseases*, **41**, 141–7.

Alto, L. E. and Dhalla, N. S. (1979). Myocardial cation contents during induction of calcium paradox. *American Journal of Physiology*, **237** (*Heart Circulation Physiology*, **6**), H713–19.

Anderson, D., Braughler, J., Hall, E., Waters, T., McCall, J., and Means, E. (1988). Effects of treatment with U74006F on neurological outcome following experimental spinal cord injury. *Journal of Neurosurgery*, **69**, 562–7.

Anderson, D. K., Means, E. D., and Waters, T. R. (1980*a*). Spinal cord energy metabolism in normal and post laminectomy cats. *Journal of Neurosurgery*, **52**, 387–91.

Anderson, D. K., Means, E. D., Waters, T. R., and Green, B. S. (1980*b*). Spinal cord energy metabolism following compression trauma to the feline spinal cord. *Journal of Neurosurgery*, **53**, 375–80.

Anderson, D. K., Prockop, L. D., Means, E. D., and Hartley, L. E. (1976). Cerebrospinal fluid lactate and electrolyte levels following experimental spinal cord injury. *Journal of Neurosurgery*, **44**, 715–22.

Anderson, D. K., Means, E. D., Walters, T. R., and Green, B. S. (1982). Microvascular perfusion and metabolism in injured spinal cord after methylprednisolone treatment. *Journal of Neurosurgery*, **56**, 106–13.

Anderson, D. K., Saunders, R. D., Demediuk, P., Dugan, L. L., Braughler, J. M., Hall, E. D. *et al.* (1985). Lipid hydrolysis and peroxidation in injured spinal cord: partial protection with methylprednisolone or vitamin E and selenium. *Central Nervous System Trauma*, **2**, 257–67.

Arias, M. J. (1987). Treatment of experimental spinal cord injury with TRH, naloxone, and dexamethasone. *Surgical Neurology*, **28**, 335–8.

Ashraf, M. (1987). Oxygen derived radicals related injury in the heart during calcium paradox. *Virchows Archiv* [B], **54**(1), 27–37.

Ashraf, M., Onda, M., Hirohata, Y., and Schwartz, A. (1982). Therapeutic effect of diltiazem on myocardial cell injury during the calcium paradox. *Journal of Molecular and Cellular Cardiology*, **14**(6), 323–7.

Baker, J. E. and Hearse, D. J. (1983*a*). Slow calcium channel blockers and the calcium paradox: comparative studies in the rat with seven drugs. *Journal of Molecular and Cellular Cardiology*, **15**, 475–85.

Baker, J. E. and Hearse, D. J. (1983*b*). The temperature-sensitivity of slow channel calcium blockers in relation to their effect upon the calcium paradox. *European Heart Journal*, **4**, (Suppl. H), 97–103.

Baker, J. E. and Hearse, D. J. (1985). Differing potencies and dose–response characteristics in the ability of slow-calcium-channel blockers to reduce enzyme leakage in the calcium paradox. *Advanced Myocardiology*, **6**(1985), 637–46.

Baker, J. E., Bullock, G. R., and Hearse, D. J. (1983). The temperature dependence of the calcium paradox: enzymatic, functional, and morphological correlates of cellular injury. *Journal of Molecular and Cellular Cardiology*, **15**, 393–411.

Baker, J. E., Kemmenoe, B. H., Hearse, D. J., and Bullock, G. R. (1984). Calcium delivery and time: factors affecting the progression of cellular damage during the calcium paradox in the rat heart. *Cardiovascular Research*, **18**, 361–70.

Balentine, J. D. (1978*a*). Pathology of experimental spinal cord trauma I. The necrotic lesion as a function of vascular injury. *Laboratory Investigation*, **39**, 236–53.

Balentine, J. D. (1978*b*). Pathology of experimental spinal cord trauma. II. Ultrastructure of axons and myelin. *Laboratory Investigation*, **39**, 254–5.

Balentine, J. D. (1983). Calcium toxicity as a factor in spinal cord injury. *Surveys and Syntheses of Pathological Research*, **2**, 184–93.

Balentine, J. D. and Dean, D. (1982). Calcium-induced spongiform and necrotizing myelopathy. *Laboratory Investigation*, **47**, 286–95.

Balentine, J. D. and Green, W. B. (1984). Ultrastructural pathology of nerve fibers in calcium-induced myelopathy. *Journal of Neuropathology and Experimental Neurology*, **43**, 500–10.

Balentine, J. D. and Hilton, C. W. (1980). Ultrastructural pathology of axons and myelin in calcium induced myelopathy. *Journal of Neuropathology and Experimental Neurology*, **39**, 339–45.

Balentine, J. D. and Spector, M. (1977). Calcification of axons in experimental spinal cord trauma. *Annals of Neurology*, **2**, 520–3.

Borgens, R. B., Blight, A. R., and Murphy, D. J. (1986*a*). Axonal regeneration in spinal cord injury: a perspective and new technique. *Journal of Comparative Neurology*, **250**, 157–67.

Borgens, R. B., Blight, A. R., Murphy, D. J., and Stewart, L. (1986*b*). Transected dorsal column axons within the guinea pig spinal cord regenerate in the presence of an applied electric field. *Journal of Comparative Neurology*, **250**, 168–80.

Borgens, R. B., Blight, A. R., and McGinnis, M. E. (1987). Behavioral recovery induced by applied electric fields after spinal cord hemisection in guinea pig. *Science*, **238**, 367–9.

Bracken, M. B., Collins, W. F., Freeman, D. F., *et al.* (1984). Efficacy of methylprednisolone in acute spinal cord injury. *Journal of American Medical Association*, **251**, 45–52.

Bracken, M. B., Shepard, M. J., Hellenbrand, K. G., Collins, W. F., Leo, L. S., Freeman, D. E., *et al.* (1985). Methyprednisolone and neurological function 1 year after spinal cord injury. *Journal of Neurosurgery*, **63**, 704–13.

Bracken, M. B., Shepard, M. J., Collins, W. F., Holford, T. R., Young, W., Baskin, D. S., *et al.* (1990). A randomized controlled trial of methylprednisolone or naloxone in the treatment of acute spinal-cord injury: results of the Second National Acute Spinal Cord Injury Study. *New England Journal of Medicine*, **322**, 1405–11.

Braughler, J. M. and Hall, E. D. (1981*a*). Acute enhancement of spinal cord synaptosomal (Na$^+$-K$^+$)-ATPase activity in cats following intravenous methylprednisolone. *Brain Research*, **219**, 464–9.

Braughler, J. M. and Hall, E. D. (1981*b*). Correlation of methylprednisolone pharmacokinetics in cat spinal cord with its effect on (Na+-K+)-ATPase, lipid peroxidation and motor neuron function. *Journal of Neurosurgery*, **56**, 838–44.

Braughler, J. M. and Hall, E. D. (1982). Pharmacokinetics of methylprednisolone in cat plasma and spinal cord following a single intravenous dose of the sodium succinate ester. *Drug Metab. Dispos.*, **10**(5), 551–2.

Braughler, J. M. and Hall, E. D. (1983*a*). Lactate and pyruvate metabolism in injured cat spinal cord before and after a single large intravenous dose of methylprednisolone. *Journal of Neurosurgery*, **59**(2), 256–61.

Braughler, J. M. and Hall, E. D. (1983*b*). Uptake and elimination of methylprednisolone from contused cat spinal cord following intravenous injection of the sodium succinate ester. *Journal of Neurosurgery*, **58**(4), 538–42.

Braughler, J. M. and Hall, E. D. (1984). Effects of multi-dose methylprednisolone sodium succinate administration on injured cat spinal cord neurofilament degradation and energy metabolism. *Journal of Neurosurgery*, **61**(2), 290–5.

Braughler, J. M. and Hall, E. D. (1985). Current application of 'high-dose' steroid therapy for CNS injury. A pharmacological perspective. *Journal of Neurosurgery*, **62**(6), 806–10.

Braughler, J. M., Duncan, L. A., and Chase, R. L. (1985*a*). Interaction of lipid peroxidation and calcium in the pathogenesis of neuronal injury. *Central Nervous System Trauma*, **2**, 269–83.

Braughler, J. M., Duncan, I. A., and Goodman, T. (1985*b*). Calcium enhances *in vitro* free radical-induced damage to brain synaptosomes, mitochondria, and cultured spinal cord neurons. *Journal of Neurochemistry*, **45**, 1288–93.

Braughler, J. M., Hall, E. D., Means, E. D., Waters, T. R., and Anderson, D. K. (1987). Evaluation of an intensive methylprednisolone sodium succinate dosing regimen in experimental spinal cord injury. *Journal of Neurosurgery*, **67**(1), 102–5.

Braughler, J. M., and Hall, E. D. (1989). Central nervous system trauma and stroke. I. Biochemical considerations for oxygen radical formation and lipid peroxidation. *Free Radical Biology and Medicine*, **6**, 289–301.

Breasted, J. H. (1930). *The Edwin Smith Papyrus*, Vols I and II. University of Chicago Press.

Brown, W. E. (1971). Solubilities of phosphates and other sparingly soluble compounds. In *Environmental phosphorus handbook* (ed. E. J. Griffith, A. Beeton, J. M. Spencer, and D. T. Mitchell), pp. 203–40. Wiley, New York.

Busselen, P. (1982). The effect of potassium depolarization on the sodium dependent calcium efflux from goldfish heart ventricles and guinea pig atria. *Journal of Physiology*,

Busselen, P. (1985). Suppression of cellular injury during the calcium paradox in rat heart by factors which reduce calcium uptake by mitochondria. *Pflugers Archiv*, **404**(20), 166–71.

Busselen, P. (1987). Effects of sodium on the calcium paradox in rat hearts. *Pflugers Archiv*, **408**(5), 458–64.

Campbell, J. B., DeCrescito, V., Tomasula, J. J., Demopoulos, H. B., Flamm, E. S., and Ortega, B. D. (1974). Effect of antifibrinolytic and steroid therapy on contused cords of cats. *Journal of Neurosurgery*, **55**, 726–33.

Cawthon, D. F., Senter, H. J., and Stewart, W. B. (1980). Comparison of hydrogen clearance and 14C-antipyrine autoradiography in the measurement of spinal cord blood flow after severe impact injury. *Journal of Neurosurgery*, **37**, 591–6.

Chan, P. H. and Fishman, R. A. (1980*a*). Brain edema: induction in cortical slices by polyunsaturated fatty acids. *Science*, **201**, 358–60.

Chan, P. H. and Fishman, R. A. (1980*b*). Transient formation of superoxide radicals in polyunsaturated fatty acids-induced brain swelling. *Journal of Neurochemistry*, **35**, 1004–7.

Chan, P. H. and Fishman, R. A. (1985). Brain edema. In *Handbook of neurochemistry* (ed. A. Lajtha), Vol. 10, pp. 153–74. Plenum Press, New York.

Chan, P. H., Fishman, R. A., Caronna, J., Schmidley, J. W., Prioleau, G., and Lee, J. (1983). Induction of brain edema following intracerebral injection of arachidonic acid. *Annals of Neurology*, **13**, 625–32.

Chan, P. H., Schmidley, J. W., Fishman, R., and Langar, S. M. (1984). Brain injury edema and vascular permeability changes induced by oxygen-derived free radicals. *Neurology*, **34**, 315–20.

Chance, B. (1965). The energy-linked reaction of calcium with mitochondria. *Journal of Biological Chemistry*, **240**, 2729–48.

Chapman, R. A., Rodrigo, G. C., Tunstall, J., Yates, R. J. and Busselen, P. (1984). Calcium paradox of the heart: a role for intracellular sodium ions. *American Journal of Physiology*, **247**, H874–9.

Chapman, R. A., Fozzard, H. A., Friedlander, I. R., and January, C. T. (1986). Effects of Ca^{2+}, Mg^{2+} removal on aiNa, aiK, and tension in cardiac Purkinje fibers. *American Journal of Physiology*, **251**, C920–7.

Chughtai, A. R., Marshall, R., and Nancollas, G. H. (1968). Complexes in calcium phosphate solutions. *Journal of Physical Chemistry*, **72**, 208–11.

Demediuk, P., Saunders, R. D., Anderson, D. K., Means, E. D., and Horrocks, L. A. (1985). Membrane lipid changes in laminectomized and traumatized cat spinal cord. *Proceedings of the National Academy of Sciences of the USA*, **82**, 7071–5.

Demopoulos, H. B., Flamm, E. S., Pietronigro, D. D., Seligman, M. C., Tomasula, J., and DeCrescito, V. (1980). The free radical pathology and the microcirculation in the major central nervous system disorders. *Acta Physiologica Scandinavica*, **492**, 91–119.

Demopoulos, H. B., Flamm, E. S., Seligman, M. C., Pietronigro, D. D., Tomasula, J., and DeCrescito, V. (1981). Further studies on free radical pathology in the major central nervous system disorders: effect of very high doses of methylprednisolone on the functional outcome, morphology and chemistry of experimental spinal cord impact injury. *Canadian Journal of Physiological Pharmacology*, **60**, 1415–24.

Dohrmann, G. J., Wick, K. M., and Bucy, P. C. (1973). Spinal cord blood flow patterns in experimental traumatic paraplegia. *Journal of Neurosurgery*, **38**, 52–8.

Dow-Edwards, D., DeCrescito, V., Tomasula, J. J., and Flamm, E. S. (1982). Effect of aminophyllin and isoproterenol on spinal cord blood flow after impact injury. *Journal of Neurosurgery*, **56**, 350–8.

Ducker, T. B. and Assenmacher, D. R. (1969). Microvascular response to experimental spinal cord trauma. *Surgical Forum*, **20**, 428–30.

Ducker, T. B. and Perot, P. L. (1971). Spinal cord oxygen and blood flow in trauma. *Surgical Forum*, **22**, 413–15.

Ducker, T. B., Kindt, G. W., and Kempe, L. G. (1971). Pathological findings in acute spinal cord injury. *Journal of Neurosurgery*, **35**, 700–9.

Eichelberg, D., Peters, R., and Schmutzler, W. (1984). Recognition of the 'calcium paradox' and the effects of verapamil and gallopamil in human adenoidal mast cells. *Agents' Actions*, **14**(3–4), 410–13.

Faden, A. I. (1984). Opiate antagonists and thyrotropin-releasing hormone. II. Potential role in the treatment of central nervous system injury. *Journal of the American Medical Association*, **252**, 1452–4.

Faden, A. I. and Holaday, J. W. (1979). Opiate antagonists: a role in treatment of hypovolemic shock. *Science*, **205**, 317–18.

Faden, A. I. and Jacobs, T. P. (1985). Opiate antagonist WIN 44,441–3 stereospecifically improves neurologic recovery after ischemic spinal injury. *Neurology*, **35**, 1311–15.

Faden, A. I., Jacobs, T. P., and Holaday, J. W. (1980). Opiate antagonist improves neurologic recovery after spinal injury. *Science*, **211**, 493–4.

Faden, A. I., Jacobs, T. P., and Holaday, J. W. (1981a). Thyrotropin releasing hormone improves neurologic recovery after spinal trauma in cats. *New England Journal of Medicine*, **305**, 1063–7.

Faden, A. I., Jacobs, T. P., Mougey, E., and Holaday, J. W. (1981b). Endorphins in experimental spinal injury: therapeutic effect of naloxone. *Annals of Neurology*, **10**, 326–32.

Faden, A. I., Hallenbeck, J. M., and Brown, C. Q. (1982a). Treatment of experimental stroke: comparison of naloxone and thyrotropic releasing hormone. *Neurology (NY)*, **32**, 1083–7.

Faden, A. I., Jacobs, T. P., and Holaday, J. W. (1982b). Comparison of early and late naloxone treatment in experimental spinal injury. *Neurology (NY)*, **32**, 677–81.

Faden, A. I., Jacobs, T. P., Smith, G. P., Green, B., and Zivin, J. A. (1983a). Neuropeptides in spinal cord injury: comparative experimental models. *Peptides*, **4**, 631–4.

Faden, A. I., Jacobs, T. P., and Smith, M. T. (1983*b*). Comparison of thyrotropin-releasing hormone (TRH), naloxone, and dexamethasone treatments in experimental spinal injury. *Neurology*, **33**, 673–8.

Faden, A. I., Jacobs, T. P., and Zivin, J. A. (1983*c*). Naloxone but not a delta antagonist improves neurological recovery after spinal stroke in the rabbit. *Life Science*, **33** (Supplement 1), 707–10.

Faden, A. I., Jacobs, T. P., Patrick, D.H., and Smith, M. T. (1984*a*). Megadose corticosteroid therapy following experimental traumatic spinal injury. *Journal of Neurosurgery*, **60**, 712–17.

Faden, A. I., Jacobs, T. P., and Smith, M. T. (1984*b*). Thyrotropin-releasing hormone in experimental spinal injury: dose response and late treatment. *Neurology*, **34**, 1280–4.

Feuerstein, G., Feuerstein, N., and Hallenbeck, J. (1987). Cellular and humoral interactions in acute microvascular injury: a pivotal role for the endothelial cell. *Critical Care Medicine*, **8**, 99–118.

Flamm, E. S., Young, W., Demopoulos, H. B., DeCrescito, V., and Tomasula, J. J. (1982). Experimental spinal cord injury: treatment with naloxone. *Neurosurgery*, **10**, 227–31.

Flamm, E. S., Young, W., Collins, W. E., Piepmeier, J., Clifton, G. L., and Fischer, B. (1985). A phase I trial of nalaxone treatment in acute spinal cord injury. *Journal of Neurosrugery*, **63**, 390–7.

Ganote, C. E. and Sims, M. A. (1984). Parallel temperature dependence of contracture-associated enzyme release due to anoxia, 2,4-dinitrophenol (DNP), or caffeine and the calcium paradox. *American Journal of Physiology*, **116**, 94–106.

Goodkin, R. and Campbell, J. B. (1969). Sequential pathological changes in spinal cord injury. *Surgical Forum*, **20**, 430–2.

Greisman, S. E. (1982). Experimental gram-negative bacterial sepsis: optimal methyl-prednisolone requirements for prevention of mortality not preventable by antibiotics alone (41455). *Proceedings of the Society for Experimental Biological Medicine*, **170**, 436—42.

Grinwald, P. M. (1982). Calcium uptake during post-ischemic perfusion in the isolated rat heart: influence of extracellular sodium. *Journal of Molecular and Cellular Cardiology*, **14**, 359–65.

Gruner, J. A., Young, W., and DeCrescito, V. (1984). The vestibulospinal free fall response: a test of descending function in spinal injured cats. *Central Nervous System Trauma*, **1**, 139–60.

Guha, A., Tator, C. H., and Piper, I. (1985). Increase in rat spinal cord blood flow with the calcium channel blocker nimodipine. *Journal of Neurosurgery*, **63**, 250–9.

Guha, A., Tator, C. H., and Piper, I. (1987*a*). Effect of a calcium channel blocker on posttraumatic spinal cord blood flow. *Journal of Neurosurgery*, **66**, 423–30.

Guha, A., Tator, C. H., Endrenyi, L., and Piper, I. (1987*b*). Decompression of the spinal cord improves recovery after acute experimental spinal cord compression injury. *Paraplegia*, **25**, 324–39.

Haghighi, S. S. and Chehrazi, B. (1987). Effect of naloxone in experimental acute spinal cord injury. *Neurosurgery*, **20**, 385–8.

Hall, E. D. (1982). Glucocorticoid effects on central nervous excitability and synaptic transmission. *International Review of Neurobiology*, **23**, 165–95.

Hall, E. D. and Braughler, J. M. (1981). Acute effects of intravenous glucocorticoid pre-treatment on the *in vitro* peroxidation of cat spinal cord tissue. *Experimental Neurology*, **72**, 321–4.

Hall, E. D. and Braughler, J. M. (1982). Effects of methylprednisolone on spinal cord lipid peroxidation and (Na^+-K^+)-ATPase activity: dose response analysis during the first hour after contusion injury in the cat. *Journal of Neurosurgery*, **57**, 247–53.

Hall, E. D. and Braughler, J. M. (1989). Central nervous system trauma and stroke. II. Physiological and pharmacological evidence for involvement of oxygen radicals and lipid peroxidation *Free Radical Biology and Medicine*, **6**, 303–13.

Hall, E. D. and Wolf, D. L. (1986). A pharmacological analysis of the pathophysiological mechanisms of posttraumatic spinal cord ischemia. *Journal of Neurosurgery*, **64**(6), 951–61.

Hall, E. D., Wolf, D. L., and Braughler, J. M. (1984). Effects of a single large dose of methylprednisolone sodium succinate on experimental posttraumatic spinal cord ischemia. Dose–response and time–action analysis. *Journal of Neurosurgery*, **61**(1), 124–30.

Hall, E. D., McCall, J. M., Chase, R. L., Yonkers, P. A., and Braughler, J. M. (1987). A nonglucocorticoid steroid analog of methylprednisolone duplicates its high-dose pharmacology in models of central nervous system trauma and neuronal membrane damage. *Journal of Pharmacology and Experimental Therapy*, **242**(1), 137–42.

Hall, E. D., Yonkers, P. A., Horan, K. L., and Braughler, J. M. (1989). Correlation between attenuation of posttraumatic spinal cord ischemia and preservation of tissue vitamin E by the 21-aminosteroid U74006F: evidence for an *in vivo* antioxidant mechanism. *Journal of Neurotrauma*, **6**, 169–76.

Happel, R. D., Smith, K. P., Banik, M. L., Powers, J. M., Hogan, E. L., and Balentine, J. D. (1981). Ca^{2+} accumulation in experimental spinal cord trauma. *Brain Research*, **211**, 476–9.

Hearse, D. J. and Baker, J. E. (1981). Verapamil and the calcium paradox: a reaffirmation. *Journal of Molecular and Cellular Cardiology*, **13**, 1087–90.

Hearse, D. J., Humphrey, S. M., and Bullock, G. R. (1978). The oxygen paradox and the calcium paradox. *Journal of Molecular and Cellular Cardiology*, **10**, 641–8.

Hess, M. L. and Manson, N. H. (1984). Molecular oxygen: friend and foe. The role of the oxygen free radical system in the calcium paradox, the oxygen paradox and ischemia/reperfusion injury. *Journal of Molecular and Cellular Cardiology*, **16**(11), 969–85.

Hirata, F., Schiffman, E., Venkatasubramanian, K., Saloman, D., and Axelrod, J. (1980). A phopholipase A_2 inhibitory protein in rabbit neutropils induced by glucocorticoids. *Proceedings of the National Academy of Sciences of the USA*, **77**, 2533–6.

Hirata, M., Fukui, H., and Shimamoto, N. (1984). Inhibition by reserpine of myocardial damage due to calcium paradox in isolated guinea pig hearts. *Japanese Journal of Pharmacology*, **36**(1), 114–17.

Hoka, S., Bosnjak, Z. I., and Kampine, J. P. (1987). Halothane inhibits calcium accumulation following myocardial ischemia and calcium paradox in guinea pig hearts. *Anesthesiology*, **67**(2), 197–202.

Holaday, J. W. and D'Amato, R. J. (1982). Naloxone or TRH fails to improve neurological deficits in gerbil models of 'stroke'. *Life Science*, **31**, 385–92.

Holaday, J. W. and Faden, A. I. (1978). Naloxone reversal of endotoxin hypotension suggests role of endorphins in shock. *Nature*, **275**, 450–1.

Holaday, J. W. and Faden, A. I. (1980). Naloxone acts at central opiate receptors to reverse hypotension, hypothermia and hypoventilation in spinal shock. *Brain Research*, **189**, 295–9.

Horrocks, L. A., Demediuk, P., Saunders, R. D., Dugan, L., Clendenon, N. R., Means, E. D. *et al.* (1985). The degradation of phospholipids, formation of metabolites of arachidonic acid, and demyelination following experimental spinal cord injury. *CNS Trauma*, **2**, 115–20.

Hosobuchi, Y., Baskin, O. S., and Wood, S. K. (1982). Reversal of induced ischemic neurologic deficit in gerbils by the opiate antagonist naloxone. *Science*, **215**, 69–71.

Hsu, C. Y., Halushka, P. V., Hogan, E. L., Banik, N. L., Lee, W. A., and Perot, P. L. (1985). Alterations of thromboxane and prostacyclin levels in experimental spinal cord injury. *Neurology*, **35**, 1003–9.

Hunt, W. G. and Willis, R. J. (1985). Calcium exposure required for full expression of injury in the calcium paradox. *Biochemistry and Biophysics Research Communications*, **126**(2), 901–4.

Julicher, R. H., Sterrenberg, L., Koomen, J. M., Bast, A., and Noordhoek, J. (1984). Evidence for lipid peroxidation during the calcium paradox in vitamin E-deficient rat heart. *Naunyn-Schmiedebergs Archiv—Pharmacologie*, **326**(1), 87–9.

Kakulas, B. A. and Bedbrook, G. M. (1969). A correlative clinicopathological study of spinal cord injury. *Proceedings of the Australian Association of Neurologists*, **6**, 123–32.

Kakulas, B. A. and Bedbrook, G. M. (1976). Pathology of injuries of the vertebral spinal cord—with emphasis on the microscopic aspects. In *Handbook of clinical neurology*, Vol. 25, *Injuries of the spine and spinal cord*, Part I (ed. P. J. Vinken and G. W. Bruyn), pp. 27–42. North-Holland, Amsterdam.

Kanaide, H., Meno, H., and Nakamura, M. (1987). Metabolic and physical changes during calcium paradox induced in the rat heart. *British Journal of Experimental Pathology*, **68**, 319–30.

Karmazyn, M. (1987). Calcium paradox-evoked release of prostacyclin and immuno-reactive leukotriene C4 from rat and guinea-pig hearts; evidence that endogenous prostaglandins inhibit leukotriene biosynthesis. *Journal of Molecular and Cellular Cardiology*, **19**, 221–30.

Kastin, A. J., Nissen, C., and Olson, R. D. (1982). Failure of MIF-1 or naloxone to reverse ischemia-induced neurological deficits in gerbils. *Pharmacology and Biochemistry of Behavior*, **17**, 1083–5.

Kontos, H. A., Wei, E. P., Ellis, E. F., Povlishock, J. T., and Dietrich, W. D. (1981). Prostaglandins in physiological and in certain pathological responses of the cerebral circulation. *Fed. Proc.*, **40**, 2326–30.

Koomen, J. M., Schevers, J. A., Noordhoek, J., and Zimmerman, A. N. (1983). Magnesium and the calcium paradox: the occurrence of 'spasmodic contractions' during $Ca^{2+}Mg^{2+}$-free perfusion of isolated rat heart. *Basic Research in Cardiology*, **78**, 227–38.

Lohse, D. C., Senter, H. J., and Kauer, J. S. (1980). Spinal cord blood flow in experimental transient paraplegia. *Journal of Neurosurgery*, **52**, 335–45.

Long, J. B., Martinez Arizala, A., Petras, J. M., and Holaday, J. W. (1986). Endogenous opioids in spinal cord injury: a critical evaluation. *Central Nervous System Trauma*, **3**, 295–316.

McCall J. M., Braughler, J. M. and Hall, E. D. (1987). A new class of compounds for stroke and trauma: effects of 21-aminosteroids on lipid peroxidation. *Acta Anesthesiologica Belgica*, **38**, 417–20.

McIntire, T. M., Zimmerman, G. A., Satoh, K. *et al.* (1985). Cultured endothelial cells synthesize both platelet activating factor and prostacyclin in response to histamine, bradykinin and adenosine triphosphate. *Journal of Clinical Investigation*, **76**, 271.

Metz, R., Giebler, C., and Forster, W. (1980). Evidence for a direct inhibitory effect of glucocorticoids on the activity of phospholipase A_2 as a further possible mechanism of some actions of steroid anti-inflammatory drugs. *Pharmacological Research Communications*, **12**, 817–27.

Nayler, W. G., Perry, S. E., Elz, I. S., and Daly, M. J. (1984). Calcium, sodium, and the calcium paradox. *Clinical Research*, **55**, 227–37.

Oksendal, A. N. and Jynge, P. (1986). Myocardial protection by micromolar manganese in the calcium paradox and additive effects of verapamil. *Basic Reseach in Cardiology*, **81**, 581–93.

Oksendal, A. N. and Jynge, P. (1987). Tissue protection by adrenergic blockade in the calcium paradox? *Basic Research in Cardiology*, **82**(2) (1987 Mar.–Apr.), 138–45.

Oksendal, A. N., Jynge, P., Sellevoid, O. F., Rotevatn, S., and Saetersdal, T. (1985). The calcium paradox phenomenon: a flow rate volume response study of calcium-free perfusion. *Journal of Molecular and Cellular Cardiology*, **17**, 959–72.

Osterholm, J. L. (1974). The pathophysiological response in spinal cord injury. *Journal of Neurosurgery*, **40**, 5–33.

Pickard, J. D. (1981). Role of prostaglandins and arachidonic acid derivatives in the coupling of cerebral blood flow to cerebral metabolism. *Journal of Cerebral Blood Flow and Metabolism*, **1**, 361–84.

Rabkin, S. W. (1987). Effect of chlorpromazine on myocardial damage in the calcium paradox. *Journal of Cardiovascular Pharmacology*, **9**, 486–92.

Rossi, V., Brevario, F., Ghezzi, P., *et al.* (1985). Prostacyclin synthesis induced in vascular cells by interleukin 1. *Science*, **229**, 174–6.

Ruano Arroyo, G., Gerstenbluth, G., and Lakatta, E. G. (1984). 'Calcium paradox' in heart is modulated by cell sodium during the calcium-free period. *Journal of Molecular and Cellular Cardiology*, **16**, 783–93.

Rudge, M. F. and Duncan, C. J. (1984). Comparative studies on the calcium paradox in cardiac muscle: the effect of temperature on the different phases. *Comparative Biochemistry and Physiology [A]*, **79**, 393–8.

Ruigrok, T. J. (1985). Possible mechanisms involved in the development of the calcium paradox. *General Physiology and Biophysics*, **4**, 155–65.

Ruigrok, T. J. C., Burgerdijk, F. J. A., and Zimmerman, A. N. E. (1975). The calcium paradox: a reffirmation. *European Journal of Cardiology*, **3**, 59–63.

Sandler, A. N. and Tator, C. H. (1976). Review of the effects of spinal cord trauma on vessels and blood flow in the spinal cord. *Journal of Neurosurgery*, **45**, 638–46.

Saunders, R. D., Dugan, L. L., Demediuk, P., Means, E. D., Horrocks, L. A., and Anderson, D. K. (1987). Effects of methylprednosolone and the combination of alpha-tocopherol and selenium on arachidonic acid metabolism and lipid peroxidation in traumatized spinal cord tissue. *Journal of Neurochemistry*, **49**, 24–31.

Schanne, F. A., Kane, A. B., Young, E. E., and Farber, J. L. (1979). Calcium dependence of toxic cell death: a common pathway. *Science*, **206**, 700–2.

Senter, H. J. and Venes, J. L. (1978). Altered blood flow and secondary injury in experimental spinal cord trauma. *Journal of Neurosurgery*, **49**, 569–78.

Senter, H. J. and Venes, J. L. (1979). Loss of autoregulation and posttraumatic ischemia following experimental spinal cord trauma. *Journal of Neurosurgery*, **50**, 198–206.

Spiller, W. G. (1898). A microscopic study of the spinal cord in two cases of Pott's disease. *Bulletin of the Johns Hopkins Hospital*, **9**, 125–33.

Tator, C. H., Rivlin, A. S., Lewis, A. J., and Schmoll, B. (1984). Effect of acute spinal cord injury on axonal counts in the pyramidal tract of rats. *Journal of Neurosurgery*, **61**, 118–23.

Tunstall, J., Busselen, P., Rodrigo, G. C., and Chapman, R. A. (1986). Pathways for the movements of ions during calcium-free perfusion and the induction of the 'calcium paradox'. *Journal of Molecular and Cellular Cardiology*, **18**, 241–54.

Turner, D. M., Kassell, N. F., Sasaki, T., Comair, Y. G., Beck, D. O., and Boarini, D. J. (1984). High dose naloxone produces cerebral vasodilation. *Neurosurgery*, **15**, 192–7.

Wagner, F., Taslitz, N., White, R. L., and Yashon, D. (1969). Vascular phenomenon in the normal and traumatized spinal cord. *Anatomical Records*, **163**, 281.

Walker, J. G., Yates, R. R., O'Neill, J. J., and Yashon, D. (1977). Canine spinal cord energy state after experimental trauma. *Journal of Neurochemistry*, **29**, 929–32.

Walker, J. G., Yates, R. R., and Yashon, D. (1979). Regional canine spinal cord energy state after experimental trauma. *Journal of Neurochemistry*, **33**, 397–401.

Wallace, C. M. and Tator, C. H. (1986a). Failure of naloxone to improve spinal cord blood flow and cardiac output after spinal cord injury. *Neurosurgery*, **18**, 428–32.

Wallace, C. M. and Tator, C. H. (1986b). Spinal cord blood flow measured with microspheres following spinal injury in the rat. *Canadian Journal of Neurological Science*, **13**, 91–6.

Wallace, C. M. and Tator, C. H. (1987). Successful improvement of blood pressure, cardiac output, and spinal cord blood flow after experimental spinal cord injury. *Neurosurgery*, **20**, 710–15.

Wallace, C. M., Tator, C. H., and Frazee, P. (1986a). Relationship between post-traumatic ischemia and hemorrhage in the injured rat spinal cord as shown by colloidal carbon angiography. *Neurosurgery*, **18**, 433–9.

Wallace, C. M., Tator, C. H., and Lewis, A. J. (1986b). Failure of blood transfusion or naloxone to improve clinical recovery after experimental spinal cord injury. *Neurosurgery*, **19**, 489–94.

Wallace, M. C., Tator, C. H., and Gentles, W. M. (1987a). Failure of blood transfusion or naloxone to improve clinical recovery after experimental spinal cord injury. *Surgical Neurology*, **28**, 269–76.

Wallace, M. C., Tator, C. H., and Lewis, A. J. (1987b). Chronic regenerative changes in the spinal cord after cord compression injury in rats. *Surgical Neurology*, **27**, 209–19.

Wallace, M. C., Tator, C. H., and Piper, I. (1987c). Recovery of spinal cord function induced by direct current stimulation of the injured rat spinal cord. *Neurosurgery*, **20**, 787–884.

Wolfe, L. S. (1982). Eicosanoids: prostaglandins, thromboxanes, leukotrienes, and other derivatives of carbon-20 unsaturated fatty acids. *Journal of Neurochemistry*, **38**, 1–14.

Young, W. (1980). Hydrogen clearance measurement of blood flow: a review of technique and polarographic principles. *Stroke*, **11**, 552–64.

Young, W. (1981). Correlation of somatosensory evoked potentials and neurological findings in clinical spinal cord injury. In *Early management of cervical spinal injury* (ed. C. H. Tator). Raven Press, NY, pp. 53–66.

Young, W. (1985a). Blood flow, metabolic and neurophysiological mechanisms in spinal cord injury. In *Central nervous system trauma status report 1985* (ed. D. Becker and J. T. Povlishock), pp. 463–73. NIH, NINCDS.

Young, W. (1985*b*). Role of calcium in spinal cord injury. *Central Nervous System Trauma*, **2**, 109–14.

Young, W. (1986). Calcium paradox in neural injury: a hypothesis. *Central Nervous System Trauma*, **3**, 235–51.

Young, W. (1987*a*). Cellular defenses against excessive Ca entry in brain and spinal cord injury. In *Critical care—state of the art*, Vol. 8 (ed. F. B. Cerra and W. C. Shoemaker), pp. 71–98. The Society of Critical Care Medicine (251 E. Imperial Highway, Suite 480, Fullerton, CA 92635, USA).

Young, W. (1987*b*). The post-injury responses in trauma and ischemia: secondary injury or protective mechanisms. *Central Nervous System Trauma*, **4**, 27–52.

Young, W. (1988). Recovery mechanisms in spinal cord injury: implications for regenerative therapy. In *Neural regeneration and transplantation*, Vol. 6 (ed. F. J. Seil), pp. 157–69. Alan R. Liss, New York.

Young, W. and DeCrescito, V. (1986). Sodium ionic changes in injured spinal cords: mechanisms of edema (abstract). *Proceedings of the Society of Neuroscience*, **16**, 267.

Young, W. and Flamm, E. S. (1982). Effect of high dose corticosteroid therapy on blood flow, evoked potentials, and extracellular calcium in experimental spinal injury. *Journal of Neurosurgery*, **57**, 667–73.

Young, W. and Koreh, I. (1986). Potassium and calcium changes in injured spinal cords. *Brain Research*, **365**, 42–53.

Young, W. and Ransohoff, J. (1989). Acute spinal cord injuries: experimental therapy, pathophysiology mechanisms, and recovery of function. In *The cervical spine* (ed. H. Sherk), pp. 464–95. Lippincott, Philadelphia.

Young, W., DeCrescito, V., Tomasula, J., and Ho, V. (1980*a*). The role of the sympathetic nervous system in pressor responses induced by spinal injury. *Journal of Neurosurgery*, **52**, 473–81.

Young, W., Tomasula, J. J., DeCrescito, V., Flamm, E. S., and Ransohoff, J. (1980*b*). Vestibulospinal monitoring in experimental spinal trauma. *Journal of Neurosurgery*, **52**, 64–72.

Young, W., Flamm, E. S., Demopoulos, H. B., DeCrescito, V., and Tomasula, J. J. (1981). Effect of naloxone on posttraumatic ischemia in experimental spinal contusion. *Journal of Neurosurgery*, **55**, 209–19.

Young, W., DeCrescito, V., and Tomasula, J. J. (1982*a*). Effect of sympathectomy on spinal cord blood flow autoregulation and posttraumatic ischemia. *Journal of Neurosurgery*, **56**, 706–10.

Young, W., Koreh, I., Yen, V., and Lindsay, A. (1982*b*). Effects of sympathectomy on extracellular activity and blood flow in experimental spinal cord contusion. *Brain Research*, **253**, 105–13.

Young, W., Yen, V., and Blight, A. (1982*c*). Extracellular calcium activity in experimental spinal cord contusion. *Brain Research*, **253**, 115–23.

Young, W., DeCrescito, V., Flamm, E. S., Blight, A. R., and Gruner, J. A. (1988). Pharmacological treatments of acute spinal cord injury: a review of naloxone and methylprednisolone. *Clinical Neurosurgery*, **34**, 675–97.

Zimmerman, A. N. E. and Hulsmann, W. C. (1966). Paradoxical influence of calcium ions on the permeability of the cell membranes in the isolated rat heart. *Nature*, **211**, 646–7.

3

Spinal injury and spinal cord blood-flow: the effect of early treatment and local cooling

Robert R. Hansebout

Summary

The role of blood-flow in the acute spinal cord injury is controversial. Local cord cooling has been used to treat experimental spinal cord injury during the last fifteen years. It has shown beneficial effects in promoting return of function after a severe injury. Spinal cord blood-flow can be measured internally, using hydrogen polarography. Using this technique in the non-traumatized spinal cord of dogs, local cooling was found to markedly decrease the internal spinal cord blood-flow. It is therefore conceivable that, following acute trauma, cooling reduces the passage of noxious substances from blood-vessels into the cord tissues, and thereby has beneficial effects.

Sixteen patients with complete spinal cord injuries received a combination of parenteral dexamethasone by injection and local spinal cord cooling within the first few hours following injury. Fourteen of the patients were followed up for an average time of three years. Six out of the eight patients with complete cervical cord injuries showed improved function in two previously paralysed cervical root levels. Four out of 14 patients got back useful sensation in their legs and definite voluntary movements. One of these regained the ability to ambulate. Three additional patients showed return of light touch sensation in their lower extremities. Only one patient died, yielding a mortality rate of 6 per cent. These results compare favourably with other studies of local cord cooling in the literature. Such treatments appear to allow better than the expected rate of improvement compared with traditional treatments of such injuries. Further trials of early cord cooling in combination with parenteral steroids are to be encouraged.

Introduction

A severe spinal cord injury can cause immediate loss of all sensation and motor function as a result of irreversible cord damage. Many clinicians deem such patients to have a completely 'transected' spinal cord, although that is usually not the case (Benes 1968). A few patients with such injuries can retain some cord function for a few hours, but then deteriorate to complete permanent paralysis. Complete loss of function after a severe spinal cord injury can thus be immediate or delayed (Ducker and Assenmacher 1969), owing to progressive pathological changes of an auto-destructive nature (Allen 1914; Goodkin and Campbell 1969; Wagner *et al.* 1971).

After severe cord trauma pericapillary haemorrhages occur initially in the grey matter. There is then a delay in the pathological sequence, followed by progression to central haemorrhagic necrosis of the cord (Ducker and Assenmacher 1969), with involvement of the white matter at a later stage (Goodkin and Campbell 1969). Most of the cord damage has occurred within the eight hours following injury, suggesting that any treatment aimed at prevention of destruction must be undertaken soon after injury (Albin *et al.* 1969).

Newer modalities of treatment

In cases of spinal trauma most surgeons consider early cord decompression, either by closed or operative means, and spinal stabilization. Most agree that, when a patient with an incomplete cord injury is deteriorating, investigation with a view towards decompressive surgery is indicated. This is especially true when cord compression by bone or disc is suspected, or when a dislocation cannot be reduced by a closed method. Removal of cord compression by the increasingly used anterior approach, or the posterior approach, when indicated can allow dramatic improvement in some cases. There is still great controversy as to whether a patient with a complete cord injury should be operated on or not. Many surgeons avoid operation in such cases, since the results of surgery have been disappointing. Some studies suggest that decompressive surgery in itself doesn't always improve function in patients with incomplete cord injury either (Hansebout 1982).

Investigators have proposed many forms of treatment to try and arrest the progressive cord damage following injury. One early form of treatment was longitudinal myelotomy, proposed by Allen (1911) in animals. This was also performed by six other groups of investigators in animals (Hansebout 1982), and by three groups in humans (Allen 1914; Benes 1968; Wagner and Rawe 1976). While there was a 17 per cent ambulation rate in patients, there was also a 42 per cent mortality rate associated with the procedure (Hansebout 1982).

Changes in water and electrolytes occur in the injured cord. Increased water content and increased sodium and reduced potassium concentration in the tissues is significant the day following cord trauma, becomes maximal between the third and sixth days after injury, and then begins to recede by the ninth day after injury (Lewin *et al.* 1972, 1974). Such oedema, thought to be vasogenic (Goodman *et al.* 1976), begins in the grey matter and spreads to the white matter (Green and Wagner 1973). Oedema has often been invoked as a main or potentiating factor in progressive cord injury (Freeman and Wright 1953; Scarff 1960; Joyner and Freeman 1963; Ducker and Hamit 1969). It was felt that, in the face of increasing swelling within its unyielding covering, the oedematous cord might undergo 'ischaemic' transection (Albin *et al.* 1967).

Scarff (1960) recommended the use of 50 per cent glucose and water to reduce oedema. Other osmotic diuretics such as urea have also been proposed to decrease spinal cord oedema (Joyner and Freeman 1963). Since steroids have been said to reduce cerebral oedema (Rasmussen and Gulati 1962), it was logical to administer steroids after spinal cord injury. Steroids were administered in the experimental laboratory, with significant functional improvement in animals in ten experimental series (Hansebout 1982). Eight researchers felt they were of value, while two did not (Hansebout 1982). Our own studies indicated that steroids were of benefit for cord functional improvement in animals (Lewin *et al.* 1972, 1974), but that these beneficial effects might be by tissue stabilization of structural elements and the preservation of potassium (Hansebout *et al.* 1972; Lewin *et al.* 1974) rather than by reducing oedema (Lewin *et al.* 1972). Later, it was shown that such potassium loss from the injured cord tissue to the extracellular space may stop axonal transmission (Eidelberg *et al.* 1975). Bohlman (1979) reported that the functional recovery in 37 patients with cervical cord injuries on steroids was not better than in untreated patients. However, Gillingham (1976) found that treatments using steroids in patients with complete injuries allowed them to regain some useful motor function. In a large American co-operative study it was reported that steroids were of doubtful value in treating patients with spinal cord injury. However, in that study there was no control group in which no steroids were given (Bracken *et al.* 1985). The results of the second National Acute Spinal Cord Injury study, published in 1990, showed that patients given intravenous steroids within eight hours of their spinal cord injury had a significant improvement in neurological status compared with untreated groups. Benefits from treatment with steroids were observed in patients with either complete or incomplete lesions of the spinal cord. No beneficial effects were seen when steroids were given more than eight hours following the spinal injury (Bracken *et al.* 1990).

Various investigators have used other drugs, such as low-molecular-weight dextran and catecholamine blockade (Hedeman and Sil 1974); and crocetin (Gainer 1976). However, with the exception of steroids (Eidelberg *et al.* 1976), and possibly naloxone and thyrotropin-releasing hormone (Faden *et al.* 1981*a*, *b*), there has been little evidence of success in the treatment of acute spinal cord injury using pharmacological agents (Ducker *et al.* 1978*a*; Rivlin and Tator 1979). Hyperbaric oxygenation has also been used in the treatment of spinal cord lesions (Holbach *et al*. 1977), but the efficacy of such treatment in patients with complete injury remains uncertain.

Ischaemia and hypoxia (Fried and Goodkin 1971) have also been linked to the pathogenesis of progressive cord injury. Hypothermia has long been said to reduce ischaemic damage (Bigelow *et al*. 1950; Rosomoff 1959) and oedema (McQueen and Jeanes 1962) in the nervous system. Neurosurgeons have felt for many years that hypothermia has a protective effect in cerebral trauma (Fay 1945), possibly due to the reduction of metabolic activity of injured tissues (Rosomoff 1959). However, generalized hypothermia can induce cardiac arrest (Hegnauer 1959). Investigators have therefore tried selective cord cooling for the treatment of such injuries.

Negrin (1962) found that the aorta could be clamped for several minutes without neurological sequelae in dogs with a cooled spinal cord. Cord cooling at moderate temperatures causes no neurological abnormality in animals (Albin *et al*. 1963, 1968) or in man (Negrin (1966). Later, in 17 experimental series carried out in 11 laboratories, 14 studies showed local cord cooling was beneficial following a spinal cord injury, while three did not (Hansebout 1982).

Most investigators cooled the spinal cord using perfusion techniques, so the effects of the cooling itself compared with the perfusion were not known. An extradural induction method of cooling was developed in our laboratory which improved functional recovery in dogs when instituted immediately after injury (Hansebout *et al*. 1975) or even four hours after injury (Kuchner and Hansebout 1976). Similar findings were reported by Thienprasit *et al*. (1975). The administration of parenteral steroids seemed to augment the effects of local cord cooling after injury (Kuchner and Hansebout 1976).

Spinal cord blood-flow following injury

Following cord trauma there is said to be reduced blood-flow in the intrinsic arteries (Fried and Goodkin 1971), with better preservation of peripheral than central microvasculature (Fairholm and Turnbull 1971; Dow-Edwards *et al*. 1980). Haemorrhagic infarction of grey and surrounding white matter may occur within one to eight hours after the injury (Dohrmann *et al*. 1973). During this time there is decreased PO_2 content (Kelly *et al*. 1970; Ducker *et al*. 1978*b*) and increased lactate content in the injured tissues, suggesting ischaemia (Anderson *et al*. 1976). A large body of the literature suggests that microcirculatory failure and therefore ischaemia are important in the pathogenesis of cord injury (Gooding *et al*. 1976; Sandler and Tator, 1976*a*, *b*; Nemecek 1978; Rivlin and Tator 1978; Sasaki *et al*. 1978; Senter and Venes 1978; Wagner *et al*. 1978; Means *et al*. 1978; Senter and Venes 1979). Other investigators do not believe ischaemia is the main causal factor (Balentine 1975; Bingham *et al*. 1975; Kobrine and Doyle 1976; Smith *et al*.

1978; Griffiths 1978; Griffiths *et al.* 1979; Kobrine *et al.* 1979). Senter *et al.* (1979) stressed that reduced cord blood-flow after injury was important.

Local blood-flow can be measured, using hydrogen polarography (Auckland *et al.* 1964). Using this technique, Kobrine *et al.* (1975) demonstrated reduced blood-flow in the grey matter, while blood-flow in the white matter increased after cord injury. These findings have been confirmed by others (Bingham *et al.* 1975; Smith *et al.* 1978), and contradict the ischaemic theories of spinal cord injury pathogenesis. On the other hand, Senter and Venes (1978) found reduced blood-flow in the white matter after injury. Others (Means *et al.* 1978; Rivlin and Tator 1978) found decreased blood-flow throughout the entire cord after injury. Alderman *et al.* (1979) showed that the pressor response that follows acute spinal cord injury is probably not a major factor in the pathogenesis of haemorrhagic necrosis. It is of interest that therapies using hypertension and hypercarbia in experimental cord injury appear to be of no value (Hukuda *et al.* 1980).

The effect of cooling on spinal cord blood-flow

In our local cooling experiments for spinal cord injury, we found that 4 hours of cooling gave more benefit than prolonged cooling for 18 hours (Wells and Hansebout 1978). This was rather puzzling. Since local cord cooling has been found to be beneficial after trauma, it was logical to study the effects of local cooling on the normal spinal cord blood-flow (Hansebout *et al.* 1985).

After exposure of the spinal cord in anaesthetized dogs, platinum electrodes were placed proximally and distally into the substance of the cord, from a dorsal position, while two further electrodes were placed into the spinal cord from the lateral aspect. The previously described cooling saddle (Hansebout *et al.* 1975) was then placed over the dorsal aspect of the spinal cord (Fig. 3.1). The cooling saddle was maintained at about 3° Celsius. The blood-flow was measured using hydrogen polarography. The internal spinal cord blood-flow was decreased by an average of 50 per cent under the cooling saddle during cooling, and returned to its original level on rewarming. Spinal cord blood-flow internally at proximal and distal control sites was not significantly affected during cooling or rewarming. The actual temperature within the spinal cord during cooling was approximately 16° Celsius (Hansebout *et al.* 1985).

Allen in 1911, after a study of impact injury, theorized the following: 'Either there is a destruction of axis cylinders, directly consequent to the impact, or else owing to the impact there is an oedematous and haemorrhagic outpouring into the cord tissue, which by its pressure and chemical activity inhibits temporarily all conduction function or destroys permanently the spinal cord.' Smith *et al.* (1978) found increased blood-flow in the spinal cord after injury using the hydrogen clearance method. They felt that this

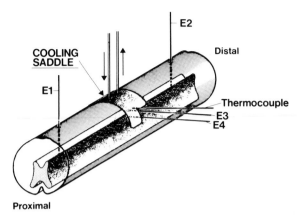

Fig. 3.1. Diagram to show the electrode placement, thermocouple, and cooling saddle. E1 and E2 were proximal and distal electrodes, while electrodes 3 and 4 were placed under the cooling saddle. (Courtesy of *Canadian Journal of Neurological Science*, **12** (1985), 84.)

'hyperaemia', if associated with breakdown of the blood–brain barrier, might secondarily injure axons by hastening oedema formation, disrupting the tissue and altering the composition of the extracellular fluid. Hypothermia to the injured nervous system has been said to exert a protective effect through a reduction of tissue metabolic requirements (Rosomoff 1959). There may be other ways through which cooling exerts beneficial effects. In the light of our most recent findings we postulate that the decreased cord blood-flow caused by cooling at an actual site of spinal cord injury tends to prevent the outpouring of oedema fluid and other toxic factors from the injured vessels, thus preserving cord function. However, if the injured cord is cooled for a prolonged time (18 hours), the beneficial effects are then eliminated, possibly as a result of the development of ischaemia enhanced by prolonged cooling. Accordingly, we felt that the maximal period of cord cooling should be 4 hours (Hansebout *et al.* 1985).

Clinical application

With the results of basic research in mind, the following clinical study was undertaken to determine the effects of restoration of function following adminstration of parenteral steroids and local cord cooling in humans with a complete sensorimotor spinal cord injury.

Equipment

A previously described apparatus (Romero-Sierra *et al*. 1974) was modified by the National Research Council of Canada (Fig. 3.2). The portable refrigeration unit consists of 16 thermo-electric cells situated under a cooling plate through which 10 per cent alcohol solution passes. A rotary pump propels the cooling fluid at 3° Celsius into a silastic saddle (Fig. 3.3) containing multiple microscopic channels. This cooling saddle rests upon the unopened dura. After passing through the saddle, the fluid is returned to the reservoir for further cooling within this closed circuit.

The cooling saddle is produced in several sizes to conform to the cervical and thoracic cord in various regions. Cooling of the cord can be done either through a posterior or an anterior approach. A thermocouple on the under-surface of the saddle monitors the temperature of the dura (Fig. 3.4).

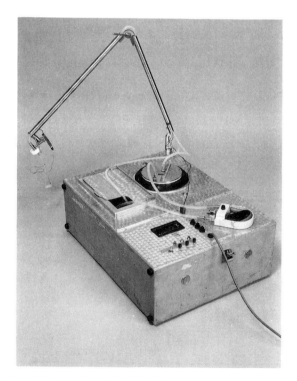

Fig. 3.2. Photograph of fifth model of cooling apparatus constructed by National Research Council of Canada. The cooling saddle is situated at the end of the boom. It can be lowered on to the dura.

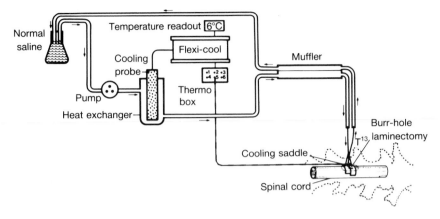

Fig. 3.3. Schematic representation of cooling circuitry and cooling saddle in the experimental laboratory. (Courtesy of *Spine*, **9** (1984), 509.)

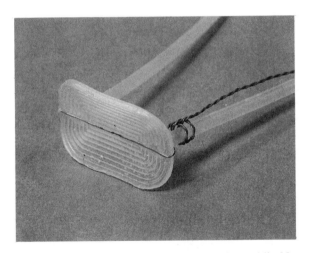

Fig. 3.4. Photograph of undersurface of spinal-cord cooling saddle. Note electrode on its undersurface to measure the dural temperature.

Methods

Our indications for cooling the cord were as follows:

1. Cooling begun 8 hours or less following the injury.
2. Complete functional neurological deficit.
3. The lesion involved the cord.
4. The patient and or relatives had given full informed consent.

On notification by a referring physician that a patient had suffered a complete spinal cord injury, we suggested a loading dose of 20 milligrams of dexamethasone be given immediately. On arrival of the patient, a general assessment was carried out to rule out multiple trauma. A complete neurological examination was done to verify completeness of the cord lesion. Absence of any sensation or voluntary motor function below the level of the lesion and an absence of reflexes, except for upgoing or slowly downgoing toes, indicated a complete lesion. Plain X-rays were then done, and in some cases a computerized transaxial tomogram. For neck injuries with a significant dislocation, cranial traction, using either tongs or a halo head-piece, was begun for attempted reduction under X-ray control. Spinal cord cooling was offered to patients who satisfied the above criteria and in whom there was no medical or surgical contraindication barring surgery.

At surgery, the spinal cord was decompressed through either an anterior or a posterior approach, whichever was indicated. A cooling saddle was placed lightly against the dura, and cooling was continued for up to 4 hours at a dural temperature of 6° Celsius. Fusion was carried out when indicated using bone in the cervical region or Harrington rods in the thoracic region by an orthopaedic surgeon. During cooling the wound was frequently irrigated, using an antibiotic solution. The wound was then closed in layers and a dressing was applied. Routine post-operative care was administered, including intermittent catheterization of the bladder and emphasizing chest physiotherapy for cervical injury cases. Dexamethasone, at 6 miligrams every 6 hours was given for 11 days, and then tapered gradually towards discontinuation on the eighteenth day after injury.

In patients with cervical injuries, arm function was evaluated from the standpoint of return of additional levels of nerve-root function compared with the immediate post-injury examination.

For all patients, both with cervical and with thoracic injuries, the motor evaluation was carried out using a modification of the scale we had previously used in animals (Hansebout *et al.* 1975) (Table 3.1). All the

Table 3.1. Motor evaluation—legs

Recovery	Grade
None	0
Flicker	1
Definite movement	2
Moderate strength	3
Strong	4
Normal	5

patients were also evaluated from the standpoint of sensory function of the legs, using a new scale we devised (Table 3.2).

Results

There were 16 patients in the series (Table 3.3). Eleven were males and five females, with a male to female ratio of 2.2 to 1. The average age for the males was 23 and that of the females 38, since one of the female patients was aged 64. The average age of all patients in the series was 27.6 years. Nine patients had cervical injuries, and seven thoracic.

   Nine of the patients had a spinal cord injury only. In addition to their cord injury, three patients had head trauma; two had head and extremity injuries; one a lacerated liver; and one a leg fracture. One patient with a severe head injury died owing to brain swelling two weeks after the accident, giving a series mortality rate of 6 per cent. Another patient experienced a cardiac arrest after surgery. During life-saving resuscitation a redislocation of the neck occurred with additional neurological loss, making subsequent evaluations difficult. That patient and the one who died were excluded from the series, leaving 14 patients who were evaluated.

Table 3.2. Sensory evaluation— legs

Recovery	Grade
None	0
Crude pressure	1
Touch	2
Above plus pain + temp. OR dorsal column	3
Above plus pain + temp. + dorsal column	4
Normal	5

Table 3.3. Characteristics of 16 patients undergoing local cord cooling

N = 16	M = 11	F = 5
M:F = 2.2:1		
Average age	M = 23	F = 38
Series average age	M + F =	27.6
Levels	C = 9	T = 7

N = number; M = males; F = female; C = cervical; T = thoracic.

The evaluation of arm function is shown in Table 3.4. Of 8 patients with cervical cord injuries, one had no recovery and one recovered one additional nerve-root level of motor function; however, 6 patients obtained an average of almost two root levels of sensory and motor functional improvement. Thus 75 per cent of the patients recovered significant sensation and motor function in their upper extremities. For a quadriplegic, two levels of motor function can be quite important.

Table 3.4. Arm recovery in 8 patients with cervical injuries—levels of nerve-root recovery

Recovery	No.	%	Sensory average	Motor average
None	1	12.5		
Sensory only	0	0.0		
Motor only	1	12.5		1.0
Sensory + Motor	6	75.0	1.7	1.7

Leg function was evaluated for all patients (Table 3.5). Those patients with thoracic cord injuries fared slightly better than those with neck injuries. Fifty per cent of the patients had no significant recovery in leg function, either sensory or motor. Three patients (21 per cent) obtained an average return of sensation to the equivalent of light touch in their lower extremities. However, 4 patients (29 per cent) recovered useful sensation in their lower extremities and, at the same time, definite voluntary motor movements. Two of these patients could extend their legs against gravity, but could not stand. One of the patients with a thoracic injury regained the ability to walk using a cane after a year, although with some spasticity and only partial return of bladder control. In considering all patients, sensory function return was of greater quality than that of motor function.

Table 3.5. Grades of recovery of leg function in 14 patients with thoracic and cervical injuries

Recovery	No.	%	Sensory grade	Motor grade
None	7	50		
Sensory only	3	21	2.00	
Sensory + Motor	4	29	3.25	1.75

The patients ranged in post-operative follow-up from one year to 70 months, with an average follow-up time of approximately three years. Fifty per cent of the patients returned to some type of employment or returned to education.

Discussion

Patients with incomplete spinal cord injuries can have a variable and unpredictable return of motor and sensory function, regardless of the type of treatment. That is not the case in those patients who have sustained a 'complete' spinal cord injury. Holdsworth (1970) and Guttmann (1973) observed that no patient with a complete loss of motor and sensory function of greater than 24 hours' duration ever walked again. There are those who argue whether patients with complete cord injuries can sometimes improve after the first few hours. In our experience, that is rarely the case. When one studies patients from the literature, approximately 1 per cent of patients with complete cervical cord injuries ever ambulate again. If one adds those patients with thoracic cord injuries, less than 2 per cent of all patients with complete cord injuries at any level ever stand or walk again. In addition, it can be shown from the literature that patients with complete cervical cord injuries have a one-year mortality rate of about 37 per cent, while any patient with a complete spinal cord injury has a one-year mortality rate of approximately 28 per cent (Hansebout 1982). Thus, to show that a new form of treatment is effective, one must improve ambulation and reduce mortality accordingly. Our results are not spectacular, but better than could be expected using conventional methods, both from the standpoint of reducing mortality and from that of promoting limb function. It appears that the combination of steroid treatment and local cooling, in our series of patients with complete cord injury, has reduced the mortality rate to about 25 per cent of that reported in other large series. In addition, the rate of ambulation has increased by a factor of about three.

In a review of the world literature, 52 patients with complete cord injuries underwent local cord cooling in other centres by various means. It is known that 35 of those patients received steroids and uncertain whether the rest did or not (Acosta-Rua 1970; Blume 1971; Selker 1971; Koons *et al.* 1972; White *et al.* 1972; Meacham and McPherson 1973; Negrin 1975; Bricolo *et al.* 1976; Tator 1979; Albin *et al.* 1980). Forty-eight per cent of those patients were considered neurologically improved, while 17 per cent of the patients became ambulatory. Seventeen per cent of the patients died. Fifty per cent of the clinicians were impressed with this form of treatment. Thus, our observations of the beneficial effects of cooling coincide with those of other observers.

In evaluating our results, one should bear in mind that preservation treatments such as cooling are applied in the experimental setting within the first 4 hours following injury. In our patients, steroids were given at an average time of about 3.25 hours following injury, while cooling was only started at an average time of 7.25 hours after injury, for technical reasons. Thus the cooling treatment was begun after most of the spinal cord damage had already occurred. This may be a limiting factor decreasing the usefulness of cooling in the clinical situation—i.e. the problem of getting the patient to the operating room on time.

The question arises as to why cooling is not used in more centres. Firstly, the equipment is not readily available everywhere. Secondly, the length of the operation is increased by several hours. Thirdly, many of the cases are injured in the middle of the night, when all personnel are not close at hand. Lastly, the results are far from spectacular, and remain somewhat controversial.

It is tempting to ask why the human does not appear to recover function as well as the laboratory animal using similar treatment. It is likely that the cord injury a patient sustains is far worse than that induced in animals under controlled conditions. In fact, many of the laboratory animals described in the literature probably had incomplete rather than complete functional cord injuries. In addition, humans suffer multiple injuries, for example, of the heart, lungs, and bones, all of which may affect the spinal cord blood supply, cause hypoxia, and also lead to the development of non-homoeostatic conditions. Some of the cord injuries in humans are well beyond the scope of any current treatment.

The role of altered blood-flow in the pathogenesis of spinal cord injury has not yet been clearly established. It is probably only one of a number of factors contributing to progressive secondary cord destruction after initial trauma. Since cooling reduces internal blood-flow and is at the same time beneficial, the situation is even more perplexing. However, since it was shown that 4 hours of cooling resulted in functional improvement, while prolonged cooling was less helpful, we confined cord cooling to 4 hours maximum. In subsequent patients with shorter follow-up, we carried out cooling only until 8 hours had elapsed since the time of the injury.

Conclusions

The addition of steroids and local cord cooling add further hope to the treatment of patients with complete spinal cord injury. It is recommended that a large dose of steroids be given as soon as possible following the injury, and continued for at least two weeks. Although the mechanism by which cooling promotes its beneficial effects is not known, its use through an extradural technique is suggested following a complete functional cord injury. However, localized cord cooling is not recommended for a period of greater than

4 hours. It is suggested that further studies be carried out utilizing a controlled series in which matched patients treated by conventional means are compared with those who receive steroids and local cord cooling. Since the efficacy of steroids and local cord cooling in the treatment of complete cord injuries has not been unequivocally established, such a study would be ethical.

Acknowledgements

I wish to thank the staff of the Montreal Neurological and Hamilton General Hospitals for their co-operation and assistance in facilitating the above trials. The cooling equipment was designed by Dr C. Romero-Sierra and built at the National Research Council of Canada, under the direction of the late Dr J. A. Tanner. The laboratory experiments were supported by Grant # MA3988 of the Medical Research Council of Canada. Support for data acquisition was provided by Spinal Cord Society (Canada).

References

Acosta-Rua, G. J. (1970). Treatment of traumatic paraplegic patients by localized cooling of the spinal cord. *Journal of the Iowa Medical Society*, **60**, 326–8.

Albin, M. S., White, R. J., and MacCarthy, C. S. (1963). Effects of sustained perfusion cooling of the subarachnoid space. *Journal of the American Society of Anaesthesiology*, **24**, 72–80.

Albin, M. S., White, R. J., Locke, G. S., Massopust, L. C., and Kretchmer, H. E. (1967). Localized spinal cord hypothermia. Anesthetic effects and application to spinal cord injury. *Anesthesia and Analgesia* (Cleveland), **46**, 8–16.

Albin, M. S., White, R. J., Acosta-Rua, G., and Yashon, D. (1968). Study of functional recovery produced by delayed localized cooling after spinal cord injury in primates. *Journal of Neurosurgery*, **29**, 113–20.

Albin, M. S., White, R. J., Yashon, D., and Harris, L. S. (1969). Effects of localized cooling on spinal cord trauma. *Journal of Trauma*, **9**, 1000–8.

Albin, M. S., Hung, T., and Babinski, M. (1980). The patient with spinal cord injury. Epidemiology, emergency and acute care: advances in physiopathology and treatment. *Current Problems in Surgery*, **17**, 190–204.

Alderman, J. L., Osterholm, J. L., D'Amore, B. R., Moberg, R. S., and Irvin, J. D. (1979). Influence of arterial blood pressure upon central hemorrhagic necrosis after severe spinal cord injury. *Neurosurgery*, **4**, 53–5.

Allen, A. R. (1911). Surgery of experimental lesion of spinal cord equivalent to crush injury or fracture dislocation of spinal column. A preliminary report. *Journal of the American Medical Association*, **57**, 878–80.

Allen, A. R. (1914). Remarks on the histopathological changes in the spinal cord due to impact. An experimental study. *Journal of Nervous and Mental Diseases*, **41**, 141–7.

Anderson, D. K., Prockop, L. D., Means, E. D., and Hartley, L. E. (1976).

Cerebrospinal fluid lactate and electrolyte levels, following experimental spinal cord injury. *Journal of Neurosurgery*, **44**, 715–22.

Auckland, K., Bower, B. F., and Berliner, R. W. (1964). Measurement of local blood flow with hydrogen gas. *Circulation Research*, **14**, 164–87.

Balentine, J. D. (1975). Central necrosis of the spinal cord induced by hyperbaric oxygen exposure. *Journal of Neurosurgery*, **43**, 150–5.

Benes, V. (1968). *Spinal cord injury*, pp. 94–6. Baillière, Tindall & Cassell, London.

Bigelow, W. G., Lindsay, W. K., and Greenwood, W. F. (1950). Hypothermia—its possible role in cardiac surgery: an investigation of factors governing survival in dogs at low body temperatures. *Annals of Surgery*, **132**, 849–66.

Bingham, W. G., Goldman, H., Friedman, S. J., Murphy, S., Yashon, D., and Hunt, W. E. (1975). Blood flow in normal and injured monkey spinal cord. *Journal of Neurosurgery*, **43**, 162–71.

Blume, H. G. (1971). *Surgical management of the cervical fracture dislocation with neurological deficit in conjunction with hypothermia of the spinal cord.* Proceedings of the 4th European Congress of Neurosurgeons, Prague, Czechoslovakia (ed. I. Fusek and Z. Kune), pp. 605–9. Czechoslovakia Medical Press, Avicenum.

Bohlman, H. H. (1979). Acute fractures and dislocations of the cervical spine. An analysis of three hundred hospitalized patients and review of the literature. *Journal of Bone Joint Surgery*, **61**(A), 1119–42.

Bracken, M. B., Shepard, M. J., Hellenbrand, K. G., Collins, W. F., Leo, L. S., Freeman, D. E., *et al.* (1985). Methylprednisolone and neurological function 1 year after spinal cord injury. Results of the National Acute Spinal Cord Injury Study. *Journal of Neurosurgery*, **63**, 704–13.

Bracken, M. B., Shepard, M. J., Collins, W. F., Holford, T. R., Young W., Baskin, D. S., *et al.* (1990). A randomized controlled trial of methylprednisolone or naloxone in the treatment of acute spinal-cord injury. *New England Journal of Medicine*, **322**, 1401–11.

Bricolo, A., Dalleore, G., Dapian, R., and Faccioli, F. (1976). Local cooling in spinal cord injury. *Surgical Neurology*, **6**, 101–6.

Dohrmann, G. J., Wick, K. M., and Bucy, P. C. (1973). Spinal cord blood flow patterns in experimental traumatic paraplegia. *Journal of Neurosurgery*, **38**, 52–8.

Dow-Edwards, D., Decrescito, V., Tomasula, J. J., and Flamm, E. S. (1980). Effect of aminophylline and isoproterenol on spinal cord blood flow after impact injury. *Journal of Neurosurgery*, **53**, 385–90.

Ducker, T. B. and Assenmacher, D. R. (1969). Microvascular response to experimental spinal cord trauma. *Surgical Forum*, **20**, 428–30.

Ducker, T. B. and Hamit, H. F. (1969). Experimental treatments of acute spinal cord injury. *Journal of Neurosurgery*, **30**, 693–7.

Ducker, T. B., Salcman, M., and Daniell, H. B. (1978*a*). Experimental spinal cord trauma III: therapeutic effect of immobilization and pharmacological agents. *Surgical Neurology*, **10**, 71–6.

Ducker, T. B., Salcman, M., Perot, P. L., and Ballantine, D. (1978*b*). Experimental spinal cord trauma I: correlation of blood flow, tissue oxygen and neurologic status in the dog. *Surgical Neurology*, **10**, 60–3.

Eidelberg, E., Sullivan, J., and Brigham, A. (1975). Immediate consequences of spinal cord injury: possible role of potassium in axonal conduction block. *Surgical Neurology*, **3**, 317–21.

Eidelberg, E., Staten, E., Watkins, C. J., and Smith, J. S. (1976). Treatment of experimental spinal cord injury in ferrets. *Surgical Neurology*, **6**, 243–6.

Faden, A. I., Jacobs, T. P., and Holaday, J. W. (1981a). Thyrotropin-releasing hormone improves neurologic recovery after spinal trauma in cats. *New England Journal of Medicine*, **305**, 1063–7.

Faden, A. I., Jacobs, T. P., Mougey, E., and Holaday, J. W. (1981b). Endorphines in experimental spinal injury: Therapeutic effect of naloxone. *Annals of Neurology*, **4**, 326–32.

Fairholm, D. J. and Turnbull, I. M. (1971). Microangiographic study of experimental spinal cord injuries. *Journal of Neurosurgery*, **35**, 277–86.

Fay, T. (1945). Observations on generalized refrigeration in cases of severe cerebral trauma. *Research in Nervous and Mental Disease*, **24**, 611–19.

Freeman, L. W. and Wright, T. W. (1953). Experimental observations of concussion and contusion of the spinal cord. *Annals of Surgery*, **137**, 433–43.

Fried, L. C. and Goodkin, R. (1971). Microangiographic observations of the experimentally traumatized spinal cord. *Journal of Neurosurgery*, **35**, 709–14.

Gainer, J. V. (jun.) (1976). Use of crocetin in experimental spinal cord injury. *Journal of Neurosurgery*, **46**, 358–60.

Gillingham, J. (1976). Early management of spinal cord trauma. Letter to the Editor (C). *Journal of Neurosurgery*, **44**, 766.

Gooding, M. R., Wilson, C. B., and Hoff, J. T. (1976). Experimental cervical myelopathy: autoradiographic studies of spinal cord blood flow patterns. *Surgical Neurology*, **5**, 233–9.

Goodkin, R. and Campbell, J. B. (1969). Sequential pathological changes in spinal cord injury: a preliminary report. *Surgical Forum*, **20**, 430–2.

Goodman, J. H., Bingham, W. G. (jun.), and Hunt, W. E. (1976). Ultrastructural blood–brain barrier alterations and edema formation in acute spinal cord trauma. *Journal of Neurosurgery*, **44**, 418–24.

Green, B. A. and Wagner, F. C. (1973). Evolution of edema in the acutely injured spinal cord. A fluorescence microscopic study. *Surgical Neurology*, **1**, 98–101.

Griffiths, I. R. (1978). Ultrastructural changes in spinal grey matter microvasculature after impact injury. *Advances in Neurology*, **20**, 415–22.

Griffiths, I. R., Trench, J. G., and Crawford, R. A. (1979). Spinal cord blood flow and conduction during experimental cord compression in normotensive and hypotensive dogs. *Journal of Neurosurgery*, **50**, 353–60.

Guttmann, L. (1973). *Spinal cord injuries*. Blackwell, London.

Hansebout, R. R. (1982). A comprehensive review of methods of improving cord recovery after acute spinal cord injury. In *Early management of acute spinal cord injury* (ed. C. H. Tator), pp. 181–96. Seminars in Neurological Surgery. Raven Press, New York.

Hansebout, R. R., Lewin, M. G., and Pappius, H. M. (1972). Evidence regarding the action of steroids in injured spinal cords. In *Steroids and brain edema* (ed. H. G. Reulen and K. Schurmann), pp. 153–6. Springer-Verlag, Berlin.

Hansebout, R. R., Kuchner, E. F., and Romero-Sierra, C. (1975). Effects of local hypothermia and of steroids upon recovery from experimental spinal cord compression injury. *Surgical Neurology*, **4**, 531–6.

Hansebout, R. R., Lamont, R. N., and Kamath, M. V. (1985). The effects of local cooling on canine spinal cord blood flow. *Canadian Journal of Neurological Sciences*, **12**, 83–7.

Hedeman, L. S. and Sil, R. (1974). Studies in experimental cord trauma. Part 2: Comparison of treatment with steroids, low molecular weight dextran and catechol-amine blockade. *Journal of Neurosurgery*, **40**, 44–51.

Hegnauer, A. H. (1959). Lethal hypothermic temperatures for dog and man. *Academy of Sciences*, **80**, 315.

Holbach, K. H., Wassmann, H., and Linke, D. (1977). The use of hyperbaric oxygena-tion in the treatment of spinal cord lesions. *European Neurology*, **16**, 213–21.

Holdsworth, F. (1970). Fractures, dislocations and fracture-dislocations of the spine. *Journal of Bone and Joint Surgery*, **52A**, 1534–51.

Hukuda, S., Mochizuki, T., and Ogata, M. (1980). Therapeutic trial of combined hypertension and hypercarbia on experimental acute spinal cord injury. *Neuro-surgery*, **6**, 644–8.

Joyner, J. and Freeman, L. W. (1963). Urea and spinal cord trauma. *Neurology (Minneapolis)*, **13**, 69–71.

Kelly, D. L., Lassiter, K. R., Calogero, J. A., and Alexander, E. (1970). Effects of local hypothermia and tissue oxygen studies in experimental paraplegia. *Journal of Neurosurgery*, **33**, 554–63.

Kobrine, A. I. and Doyle, T. F. (1976). Role of histamine in posttraumatic spinal cord hyperemia and the luxury perfusion syndrome. *Journal of Neurosurgery*, **44**, 16–20.

Kobrine, A. I., Doyle, T. F., and Martin, A. N. (1975). Local spinal cord blood flow in experimental traumatic myelopathy. *Journal of Neurosurgery*, **42**, 144–9.

Kobrine, A. I., Evans, D. E., and Rizzoli, H. V. (1979). The effects of ischemia on long-tract neural conduction in the spinal cord. *Journal of Neurosurgery*, **50**, 639–44.

Koons, D. D., Gildenberg, P. L., Dohn, D. F., and Henoch, M. (1972). Local hypo-thermia in the treatment of spinal cord injuries: Report of seven cases. *Cleveland Clinical Quarterly*, **39**, 109–17.

Kuchner, E. F. and Hansebout, R. R. (1976). Combined steroid and hypothermia treatment of experimental spinal cord injury. *Surgical Neurology*, **6**, 371–6.

Lewin, M. G., Pappius, H. M., and Hansebout, R. R. (1972). Effects of steroids on edema associated with injury of the spinal cord. In *Steroids and brain edema* (ed. H. G. Reulen and K. Schurmann), pp. 101–12. Springer-Verlag, Berlin.

Lewin, M. G., Hansebout, R. R., and Pappius, H. M. (1974). Chemical characteristics of traumatic spinal cord edema in cats. Effect of steroids on potassium depletion. *Journal of Neurosurgery*, **40**, 65–75.

McQueen, J. D. and Jeanes, L. D. (1962). Influence of hypothermia on intracranial hypertension. *Journal of Neurosurgery*, **19**, 277–88.

Meacham, W. F. and McPherson, W. F. (1973). Local hypothermia in the treatment of acute injuries of the spinal cord. *Southern Medical Journal*, **66**, 95–7.

Means, E. D., Anderson, D. K., Nicolosi, G., and Gaudsmith, J. (1978). Microvascular perfusion experimental spinal cord injury. *Surgical Neurology*, **9**, 353–9.

Negrin, J. (jun.) (1962). Prévention des lésions ischémiques de la moelle epinière par l'hypothermie régionale extravasculaire. *Revue Neurologique*, **106**, 725–9.

Negrin, J. (jun.) (1966). Local hypothermia of the spinal cord for relief of spasticity and rigidity: preliminary observations. *Archives of Physical Medicine and Rehabilitation*, **47**, 169–73.

Negrin, J. (1975). Spinal cord hypothermia: neurosurgical management of immediate and delayed post-traumatic neurologic sequelae. *New York State Journal of Medicine*, **75**, 2387–92.

Spinal injury and spinal cord blood-flow | 75

Nemecek, S. T. (1978). Morphological evidence of microcirculatory disturbances in experimental spinal cord trauma. *Advances in Neurology*, **20**, 395–405.
Rasmussen, T. and Gulati, D. R. (1962). Cortisone in the treatment of postoperative cerebral edema. *Journal of Neurosurgery*, **19**, 535–44.
Rivlin, A. S. and Tator, C. H. (1978). Regional spinal cord blood flow in rats after severe cord trauma. *Journal of Neurosurgery*, **49**, 844–53.
Rivlin, A. S. and Tator, C. H. (1979). Effect of vasodilators and myelotomy on recovery after acute spinal cord injury in rats. *Journal of Neurosurgery*, **50**, 349–52.
Romero-Sierra, C., Sierhuis, A., Hansebout, R. R., and Lewin, M. (1974). A new method for localized spinal cord cooling. *Medical and Biological Engineering*, (**March**), 188–93.
Rosomoff, H. L. (1959). Protective effects of hypothermia against pathological processes of the nervous system. *Annals of the New York Academy of Sciences*, **80**, 475–86.
Sandler, A. N. and Tator, C. H. (1976a). Effect of acute spinal cord compression injury on regional spinal cord blood flow in primates. *Journal of Neurosurgery*, **45**, 660–76.
Sandler, A. N. and Tator, C. H. (1976b). Review of the effect of spinal cord trauma on the vessels and blood flow in the spinal cord. *Journal of Neurosurgery*, **45**, 638–46.
Sasaki, S., Schneider, H., and Renz, S. (1978). Microcirculatory disturbances during the early phase following experimental spinal cord trauma in the rat. *Advances in Neurology*, **20**, 423–31.
Scarff, J. E. (1960). Injuries of the vertebral column and spinal cord. In *Injuries of the brain and spinal cord and their coverings* (4th edn) (ed. S. Brook), pp. 530–89. Springer-Verlag, Berlin.
Selker, R. G. (1971). Ice water irrigation of the spinal cord. *Surgical Forum*, **22**, 411–13.
Senter, H. J. and Venes, J. L. (1978). Altered blood flow and secondary injury in experimental spinal cord trauma. *Journal of Neurosurgery*, **49**, 569–78.
Senter, H. J. and Venes, J. L. (1979). Loss of autoregulation and posttraumatic ischemia following experimental spinal cord trauma. *Journal of Neurosurgery*, **50**, 198–206.
Senter, H. J., Venes, J. L., and Kauer, J. S. (1979). Alteration of posttraumatic ischemia in experimental spinal cord trauma by a central nervous system depressant. *Journal of Neurosurgery*, **50**, 207–16.
Smith, A. J. K., McCreery, D. B., Bloedel, J. R., and Chou, S. (1978). Hyperemia, CO_2 responsiveness, and autoregulation in the white matter following experimental spinal cord injury. *Journal of Neurosurgery*, **48**, 239–51.
Tator, C. H. (1979). Spinal cord cooling and irrigation for treatment of acute cord injury. In *Neural trauma* (ed. J. A. Popp, R. S. Bourke, L. R. Nelson, and H. K. Kimelberg), pp. 363–70. Raven Press, New York.
Thienprasit, P., Bantli, H., Bloedel, J. R., and Chou, S. N. (1975). Effect of delayed local cooling on experimental spinal cord injury. *Journal of Neurosurgery*, **42**, 150–4.
Wagner, F. C. and Rawe, S. E. (1976). Microsurgical anterior cervical myelotomy. *Surgical Neurology*, **5**, 229–31.
Wagner, F. C., Dohrmann, G. J., and Bucy, P. C. (1971). Histopathology of transitory traumatic paraplegia in the monkey. *Journal of Neurosurgery*, **35**, 272–6.
Wagner, F. C., VanGilder, J. C., and Dohrmann, G. J. (1978). Pathological changes

from acute to chronic in experimental spinal cord trauma. *Journal of Neurosurgery*, **48**, 92–8.

Wells, J. D. and Hansebout, R. R. (1978). Local hypothermia in experimental spinal cord trauma. *Surgical Neurology*, **10**, 200–4.

White, R. J., Yashon, D., Albin, M. S., and Demian, Y. K. (1972). The acute management of cervical cord trauma with quadriplegia. Presented at Annual meeting of the American Association of Neurological Surgeons, Boston, Massachusetts.

II

Specific problems

Spasticity: Introduction

L. S. Illis

Spasticity is a term which is defined in various ways. To the clinician spasticity indicates abnormally increased muscle tone, with or without other manifestations of abnormal motor function. These include loss of voluntary power and co-ordination, increased tendon reflexes, altered cutaneous reflexes, reflex irradiation, clonus, and spontaneous spasm. There is a wide variation in the presentation of spasticity, between patients and in any one patient from time to time. Fluctuations in spasticity may be spontaneous—that is, we do not know the reason for them—or in response to some stimulus, which may be a change in emotional state or take the form of internal stimuli, such as those from a distended bladder.

To the physiologist, spasticity is a motor disorder with a velocity-dependent increase in muscle tone (i.e. tonic stretch reflexes) with exaggerated monosynaptic tendon reflexes. This focuses on the stretch reflex. To the experimental anatomist, spasticity is one result of the reorganization of the intact central nervous system after a lesion.

However, to the patient the disabilities that categorize the spastic person include negative symptoms of weakness, fatiguability, and lack of dexterity, often occurring days or weeks before the onset of spasticity, and positive symptoms presumed to be due to release of segmental reflexes from higher control: flexor spasms, increased tendon jerks, decreased cutaneous reflexes, and dystonic rigidity.

Spasticity is further complicated by the fact that in patients with chronic spinal lesions, such as chronic spinal injury, the clinical features are different from those of spasticity resulting from cerebral lesions. Dimitrijevic and Nathan (1967) and Dimitrijevic, Nathan, and Sherwood (1980) have shown waxing and waning of excitability of plastic and tonic stretch reflexes, and habituation and sensitization of segmental reflexes by stimulus-induced activation of latent propriospinal inhibitory and excitatory mechanisms. In patients where the lesion results in brainstem impairment and there is preservation of ascending and descending pathways, this does not occur. Although the two groups, brainstem and spinal, share the similarity of exaggerated tendon jerks and phasic spasticity, these differences and the tonic component and the response to exteroceptive and proprioceptive stimuli are marked, and indicate that spasticity is not a single phenomenon but the complicated result of an integrated control system.

It would help if we could penetrate beneath the definitions and descriptions of spasticity and discover its pathophysiological basis in order to offer more rational treatment. For example, if spasticity, strictly defined, develops later than the negative symptoms described above then it would suggest the treatment of the spasticity would do little to influence the other lost functions. There has been slow but steady progress in the endeavour to elucidate the pathophysiological basis of spasticity. The progress is slow because many of the hypotheses of mechanisms are difficult to test in man. New physiological and other work has brought us to the point where some long-held beliefs have been refuted, and technology has developed so that hypotheses can be rigorously tested in man. Although animal experiments have provided the detailed infrastructure of knowledge of the motor system, animal models of spasticity have often been misleading.

4

Spasticity I:
Clinical aspects
L. S. Illis

The role of muscle tone in movement: anatomical considerations

Muscle possesses some elasticity, but most of the resting condition of muscle tone or tension is of reflex nature and is maintained by afferent impulses which arise in the muscle spindles. The spindles form part of a servo-mechanism signalling to the CNS information about the length of the muscle. More information which is available to central processors includes information about the speed with which lengthening occurs, and the central nervous system (spinal cord) is also able to adjust the sensitivity of the muscle spindles.

The normal resting tone is maintained by the tonic stretch reflex. On moving the limb, as in testing tone clinically, the muscle is suddenly stretched, and this elicits the phasic stretch reflex. The difference between the tonic stretch reflex and the phasic stretch reflex is due chiefly to the rapidity of stretching, and the difference between muscle tension tested by palpation and by passive stretching is probably best explained, again, by the tonic stretch versus the phasic stretch reflex. For example, in capsular hemiplegia the tone tested by palpation may be reduced, whereas tone tested by passive stretch is increased.

Gamma-loop and alpha-motor-neurons collaborate in the execution of movement, and are subject to supraspinal control. For example, clinical neurological signs of the state of tone and myotatic reflexes at the beginning and at the end of the clinical examination may show subtle differences, and are a reflection of the patient's mood and state of relaxation: unusually brisk jerks at the beginning of clinical examination are not necessarily pathological.

The organization of the spinal cord adds further understanding and further complexity to the central nervous system control, and the interaction between the gamma- and alpha-neuron systems. Not only are nerve cells organized in columnar and somato-topical arrangements, but dendrites are arranged in specific patterns. For example, some dendrites are arranged longitudinally within the cell column to which the cell belongs (Scheibel and Scheibel 1966). A single dorsal root supplying monosynaptic afferents may spread collaterals over several segments rostrally and caudally and also to contralateral dendrites (Illis 1967, 1973). In this way the effects of spindles in a single muscle may activate motor neurons in several spinal cord segments, including contralateral segments. The endings of dorsal root collaterals are different in different sites. For example up to 50 per cent of terminals on the ipsilateral cell surface are from monosynaptic afferents, whereas less than 30 per cent of terminals on ipsilateral dendrites are from dorsal root mono-synaptic afferents. On the contralateral side of the spinal cord, less than 10 per cent of terminals on cells are from crossed monosynaptic afferents, and not more than 15 per cent of terminals on dendrites are from crossed mono-synaptic afferent fibres. At least four times as many monosynaptic afferent fibres end on the ipsilateral side compared to the contralateral side (Illis 1967—in the cat spinal cord). A similar differential arrangement is valid for descending supraspinal afferents (cortico-spinal). The total effect is that of a network of a number of motor units distributed over several segments of the spinal cord supplying many different muscles giving an anatomical substrate for the functional organization of muscle tone and movement. Alteration of the substrate by a lesion alters both impulse traffic and anatomical organiza-tion (see Illis 1988), producing a change in muscle tone and power and move-ment. Since an anatomical substrate exists, the pattern of disturbance will reflect the pattern of connection. For example, cortico-spinal and rubro-spinal tracts activate flexor neurons and inhibit extensor neurons, while vestibulo-spinal activity has the opposite effect. Fibre systems end in different parts of the spinal cord: those concerned with facilitation of flexor neurons end in V–VI and dorsal VII, and those concerned with extensor facilitation end in ventral VII and VIII, ending therefore on different sets of interneurons (see Brodal 1969). This simplified view is complicated further by the fact that there are several supraspinal descending pathways within each group, and there are interactions between descending afferents in the intact spinal cord and anatomical disturbances in the partially damaged cord.

Clinical features

Evolution of spasticity in a transverse lesion of the spinal cord

In a complete lesion of the spinal cord (nearly always traumatic) there is complete paralysis and anaesthesia below the level of the lesion. Immediately after the lesion, tone is flaccid and all reflexes are absent. This is the initial stage of spinal shock, and is followed by the stage of reorganization, during which autonomous activity of the severed cord appears, with the reappearance of sweating, and of automatic reflex activity of the bladder and rectum. Later, muscles regain tone and reflexes simultaneously appear. This reorganization, which may include paraplegia in flexion, with severe spasticity, usually requires several months to evolve. Animals lower in the phylogenetic scale regain automatic and reflex behaviour more rapidly, as though the spinal reflex apparatus is more independent of descending control in lower evolutionary species. At spinal level there is a disorganization of the 'synaptic zone', which may account for the cessation and then reduction of spinal neuron excitability, with an ensuing reorganization which may explain the return of reflex activity in an altered form (Illis 1963). This clinical picture is different at different levels of cord transection, and is altered by infection or by the development of pressure sores.

In a gradually progressive partial lesion as opposed to the acute lesion described above, the evolution is different, although the final result may be the same.

Spasticity is one of the inevitable consequences of a spinal cord lesion. In man spasticity usually begins about three weeks after the lesion in both complete and incomplete disturbances (i.e. spinal shock lasts something like three weeks). However there are many exceptions to this. Spasticity tends to occur later in high cervical lesions, much earlier in some incomplete lesions, and may not occur at all where a transverse lesion is combined with a longitudinal lesion or where there are two lesions present and the lower lesion is in the cauda equina. The spasticity which is entirely secondary to the lesion itself is sometimes called 'basic spasticity', as opposed to 'excess spasticity', which is thought to be due to imposed afferent stimuli which can be prevented by appropriate management (Michaelis 1976). Michaelis suggests that the basic type of spasticity has some advantages, in that the patient may use spasticity in order to initiate emptying of automatic bladder or flexion of the leg at hip and knee. This degree of spasticity, as opposed to excess spasticity, which has considerable disadvantages and complications, rarely needs medical treatment. The major complication is the development of contractures, which appears to impose more severe spasticity, which itself increases the contracture defect. All abnormalities below the level of the spinal cord lesion are likely to increase spasticity. Such processes include constipation, infection, pressure sores or any other kind of damage, fractures, and dislocations.

Particularly in high lesions, sudden change of temperature will alter the degree of spasticity, as will physical or emotional stress.

Evolution of spasticity in lesions of the primary motor area and internal capsule

Although spasticity is usually described as being due to pyramidal lesions, and the term 'pyramidal hypertonia' is sometimes used to distinguish the increase in tone from rigidity which is of extrapyramidal origin, this is not strictly true clinically. Although the two types of increase of tone are distinct clinical entities with different clinical features it is impossible to designate a definite pathophysiology to each type, and many of the underlying mechanisms are common to both. Moreover, the term 'pyramidal hypertonia' is confusing, since lesions of the pyramidal tract do not cause hypertonia; it is para-pyramidal lesions, such as lesions of the suppressor strip area 4S, which produce hypertonia, or lesions of area 6, the para- or juxta-pyramidal area, which may be responsible.

Further levels involved in the control of muscle tone include the basal ganglia, the mid-brain, the vestibular apparatus, the spinal cord, and the neuromuscular system. The brainstem reticular formation contains both inhibitory and facilitatory areas. The cerebral cortex (suppressor strips), the basal ganglia, and the anterior lobe of the cerebellum connect with bulbar inhibitory areas. Facilitatory pathways include reticulo-spinal and vestibulo-spinal.

All the motor pathways from the primary motor area to anterior horn cells pass through the internal capsule, and the motor symptoms are similar whether the lesion is in the cortex or in the internal capsule (cortical lesions are likely to produce a monoplegia, whereas capsular lesions, where fibres are more tightly packed, tend to produce haemiplegia).

In acute lesions, flaccid paralysis with absent reflexes is present, as in the initial stage of spinal shock. Much earlier (usually a matter of hours) in spinal lesions, plantar responses appear; but tendon reflexes usually take a matter of days to return. Simultaneously, muscle tone increases with the development of spasticity, which is usually more evident in the leg than in the arm. Muscle tone is greater in extensor muscles of the leg, but tends to be more marked in the upper limb, in shoulder abductors, elbow flexors, and hand pronators. This gives the characteristic pattern seen in patients with a chronic haemiplegia, and is presumably a reflection of the pattern of endings of supraspinal pathways on interneurons.

Although some fine voluntary as well as crude flexor synergy and extensor synergy may appear (Foerster 1936) this is frequently masked by the pronounced spasticity. Improvement in spasticity may result in improved movement as described above.

Does spasticity interfere with movement?

In spastic patients the stretch reflex is altered and is hyperexcitable. Does this produce or trigger inappropriate activity? Dimitrijevic and Nathan (1967) demonstrated that antagonists may be activated, and thus produce movements opposite to those intended. McLellan (1977) showed that reflex activity may be altered by the degree of spasticity and the vigour of activity. Deterioration of performance may be produced by inappropriate activity (Pierrot-Deseilligny 1983; Corcos *et al.* 1986).

In a much earlier paper, Foerster (1936) demonstrated how spasticity may affect movement. He described in detail the problems facing a hemiplegic patient. In the legs spasticity is most developed in extensors and in the plantar flexors. Isolated dorsiflexion is opposed by the spasticity. The spasticity is of reflex nature, and can be diminished by section of some of the dorsal roots subserving plantar flexors, with the result that dorsiflexion is no longer opposed.

Treatment of spasticity

This section is not intended as a bench guide to specific treatments, and practical details of techniques and precise drug regimens and dosages are not given. This information is readily available; and in any case the doses of any particular drug will vary from patient to patient and from time to time.

One of the problems with treatment of spasticity is the difficulty in assessment and the unpredictability of pharmacological manipulation. Clinical assessment is accurate for gross changes, but is hardly susceptible to quantification. Neurophysiological assessment relies on some form of quantitative electromyography or force measurements, and the techniques are not universally accepted or applied. The neuropharmacological problem is best summed up by the fact that there are several neurotransmitters identified, but only one disease in which the responsible neurotransmitter has been established (dopamine depletion).

The primary aim of treatment is to prevent spasticity occurring, or to keep it within tolerable limits. Michaelis's (1976) concepts of basic and excess spasticity are useful in this context, as mentioned above. Basic spasticity shows little or no wasting of muscles, helps to prevent secondary complications such as osteoporosis, and is useful in triggering emptying of bladder or flexion of knee and ankle joints. By contrast, excess spasticity is *excessive*, and is due to superimposed stimuli such as those produced by contractures.

General management

Poor positioning of the limbs or failure of treatment with passive movements *from the onset of paralysis* will result in semi-fixed flexion or, less commonly, extension contractures which will increase spasticity; and this will, in turn, increase the contracture deformities. Relatively simple physiotherapeutic manœuvres will prevent this complication. The development of contractures is the most important contributory factor to excess spasticity; but any pathological process resulting, in effect, in an increase in afferent stimulation below the level of the lesion is likely to alter basic spasticity to excess spasticity. These factors include constipation, pressure sores, burns, any skin disease, urinary tract infection, unrecognized fractures or dislocations, sudden alteration of temperature or humidity and mental or physical stress. Removal or prevention of the causes of excess spasticity must precede any specific treatment.

Spasms are a serious obstacle to rehabilitation, particularly because they are often so uncontrollable. Severe spasm occurs in about one-third of patients with spinal injury, and is not unusual in the late stages of multiple sclerosis.

Preventing the progression of spasticity to a degree which would produce secondary handicaps in terms of immobility of joints, with severe postural changes, is as important, if not more important, than any other therapeutic technique.

Physical therapy

Physiotherapy: The aim of physiotherapy is to reduce spasticity and to improve voluntary motor control as a result. Increased afferent stimulation and active movement almost certainly brings inhibitory systems into action, and hopefully this will result in the better understanding of physiotherapy as a preventive and as a therapeutic measure. Several programmes for physiotherapy have been elaborated which include the elicitation of stretch reflexes, and inhibition and reciprocal inhibition of antagonist reflexes, often with marked improvement. However, in severe cases physiotherapy by itself is unlikely to succeed.

Cryotherapy: Cryotherapy or ice-therapy or cooling therapy is a technique in which ice-packs are used, and this probably produces depression of stretch reflexes. This may be beneficial when applied before physiotherapy.

Drug treatment

There are innumerable drugs which are not only useless but may be addictive (opiates) or have unacceptable side-effects (for example, chlorpromazine), or are potentially harmful. The first drug to be of real value was diazepam:

DIAZEPAM: This is a member of the benzodiazepine group widely used as tranquillizers and sedatives and, to a less extent, as anti-convulsants. Neurophysiological effects include inhibition of brainstem-activating systems (Przybyla and Wang 1968), increase in pre-synaptic inhibition (Stratten and Barnes 1971), suppression of polysynaptic spinal reflexes, and inhibition of fusimotor firing (Brausch *et al.* 1973).

Clinically, diazepam alleviates both spasticity and flexor spasms, probably by reducing abnormal excitation in antagonists (Pinelli 1973); and, since benefit is seen in complete lesions (Cook and Nathan 1967), the therapeutic action must be at spinal level. If the beneficial effect is produced by reducing abnormal excitation, then this gives further weight to the concept of excess versus basic spasticity.

BACLOFEN: This drug is a derivative of GABA, a neuro-transmitter acting predominantly at inhibitory synapses. GABA itself is not effective, since it cannot cross the blood–brain barrier. It has been shown to decrease experimental spasticity, and to be effective in man (see, for example, Sachais *et al.* 1977). It may act by inhibiting alpha-motor-neurons and fusi-motor-neurons, or facilitate Renshaw feedback inhibition. There appears to be a selective reduction in excitability of the monosynaptic reflex arc (McLellan 1973) and a decrease in substance P release or a blocking of take-up by post-synaptic receptors (Kato *et al.* 1978). An interesting effect is the report of improvement of bladder function (Jones 1971).

DANTROLENE: This appears to act distally to the neuro-muscular junction, probably by interfering with calcium ion release from the sarcoplasmic reticulum. In addition it suppresses the excitation of primary muscle spindle afferents. The effect of dantrolene as a relaxant of muscle is seen in both fast and slow muscle fibres.

Intrathecal drug treatment

The technique of intrathecal administration of drugs via a catheter connected to a reservoir and pump has been in use since about 1981, when it was first employed to relieve intractable pain (see Penn and Kroin 1987). It is clear that spinal cord processes may be pharmacologically manipulated by this method. Drugs such as morphine, clonidine, and baclofen have been used, and have been shown to have an effect on pain and spasticity and bladder function. Presumably this is via an action on specific receptors in the dorsal horn of the spinal cord, leading to alteration in spinal modulatory systems and central sensory transmission and processing. Examples of such pharmacological manipulation include enhancement of flexor reflexes by intrathecal noradrenalin (Dhawan and Sharma 1970), enhancement of Renshaw recurrent inhibition (Roby *et al.* 1981), alteration in polysynaptic flexor reflex activity (Willer and Bussel 1980), and suppression of spasticity (Struppler *et al.* 1985; Erickson *et al.* 1985). Bolus doses of morphine cause naloxone reversible alterations in bladder function and spasticity (Herman *et al.* 1988; Wainberg *et al.* 1987).

Direct infusion of drugs into the subarachnoid space of the CSF prevents problems encountered by systemic administration. For example, severe side-effects, peripheral drug deactivation, impaired drug absorption, protein binding, inadequate penetration of the blood–brain barrier, and poor patient compliance are all reduced by intrathecal drug delivery systems.

The extent of penetration of the drug into the nervous system depends on a number of factors, including the agent to be used and the method of administration. Bolus injections into the subarachnoid initially result in high CSF drug concentration and relatively limited parenchymal penetration. Serial bolus injections of low concentration of an agent are more effective and less toxic than a single large dose; but for longer-duration action and deeper diffusion into the parenchyma (for example, the ventral horn) continuous infusion is necessary, and the pharmacological agent is then concentrated at the site which is presumed to be the anatomical location of the sensory processes which subserve enhanced somatic reflexes (spasticity) and autonomic reflexes (detrusor hyperactivity).

When neurotransmitters or their agonists or precursors are applied in this way the neurological action is limited to that particular region. That is, there is little direct distribution to higher levels of the CNS. The duration of action and the clinical effectiveness of any particular drug is due, in part, to the efficiency of the drug–receptor interaction. As metabolism makes a relatively minor contribution, the rate at which drugs are redistributed into the peripheral circulation would be a limiting factor, and this is largely dependent on the lipid solubility coefficient of the agent and the binding capacity once it is within the tissue. Drugs with a low lipid solubility, for example neuropeptides, will produce a behavioural effect at concentrations which are virtually inactive systematically. They are also much better candidates for deeper parenchymal penetration than pharmacological agents which readily cross the blood–brain barrier.

It is likely that intrathecal drug-delivery systems will be the most effective way of treating spasticity, and may well have other beneficial effects, such as suppression of pain and improvement of bladder function.

Chemical interruption of the reflex arc

If the reflex arc is interrupted then spasticity can no longer be a clinical manifestation. Direct interruption by the local injection of toxic substances may be carried out at the motor point, the nerve, the nerve root at or near the root exit, subarachnoid or intrathecal injection, affecting several nerve roots, or in the spinal cord.

PROCAINE: Procaine is used for short-acting effects, such as localizing the site of subsequent injections.

PHENOL AND ALCOHOL: These are used for long-acting or possibly permanent interruption of the reflex arc. Nathan (1959) introduced phenol injections in the belief that injection produces destruction of small nerve-fibres, and thus a selective reduction in fusimotor activity. In a later paper (Nathan 1965) he suggested that in fact phenol destroys nerve-fibres in a non-selective manner. Phenol probably produces its effect by decreasing afferent bombardment to the spinal segmental neurons, and thereby reducing excessive motor neuron activity, and allowing latent patterns of co-ordination to emerge.

These substances, introduced as for lumbar puncture, with the patient adjusted to insure that the solution collects in the area of the appropriate nerve root, may reduce spasticity for many years. The technique should only be used where other methods of treatment have failed, and where no spontaneous improvement is likely to occur. Contractures are unlikely to benefit, and there is a risk of producing incontinence in patients who previously had intact sphincters. The increased sensory deficit raises the risk of pressure sores and constipation. Bladder automatism and potency may be abolished, and it is clear that these blocks are only indicated as an ultimate treatment.

Surgical treatment

Effective early medical treatment has resulted in a considerable decrease in surgery for spasticity, and probably only about 1–2 per cent of patients need surgical procedures.

Rhizotomy: This technique can be carried out by surgical means or by radio frequency or chemical methods. In the early part of this century Foerster (1911) described section of the posterior roots, and for many years this was the only partially effective procedure for the treatment of spasticity. Spasticity usually recurred eventually. A refinement of this technique is to use intraoperative stimulation to define those roots which are responsible for the spasticity. The aim of this was to try to avoid the complete loss of muscle tone and, therefore, to spare some of the useful spasticity. Another variation is by producing a DREZ (dorsal root entry zone) lesion.

Chemical rhizotomy depends on the use of either alcohol or phenol, and has been discussed above.

Myelotomy: The rationale here is the interruption of spinal reflex pathways by separating the anterior horn from the posterior horn of the spinal cord. The operation is now rarely performed. It can only be carried out for paraplegic patients with no voluntary movement and no bladder function. A variety is longitudinal myelotomy as opposed to transverse myelotomy.

Orthopaedic treatment: These procedures are not so much involved in the treatment of spasticity as in the treatment or prevention of complications and bony deformation caused by spasticity. Results are likely to be unfavourable unless the imbalance of muscular tone has been treated, since if severe spasticity persists then the results of surgery will be destroyed. The aims of surgery are to prevent or correct deformity, or to stabilize or to remove any specific handicap to rehabilitation. Procedures include tenotomy, Achilles tendon lengthening, myotomy, muscle slides, and capsulotomy. In addition, bony protuberances or abnormal ossification may be removed.

Neuromuscular stimulation

Neuromuscular stimulation may be used in spastic conditions. This is a technique using surface stimulation with electrodes placed over the belly of the muscle (cathode distally placed). The strength of the stimulus used must be below that which would elicit hypertonia or spasms. Spasticity may respond to stimulation of affected muscles or of cutaneous nerves usually at 20 to 50Hz for up to 20 minutes twice a day until skin tolerance has developed. If spasticity is severe then stimulation may be gradually increased up to three hours two or three times per day (Bajd *et al.* 1985; Dimitrijević *et al.* 1987).

Spinal cord stimulation

Spinal cord stimulation was first used to treat intractable pain in 1967 as a direct application of Melzack and Wall's gate-control theory of pain (Melzack and Wall 1965). Since that time spinal cord stimulation has been used by a number of workers in more than 30 groups (Sherwood 1985).

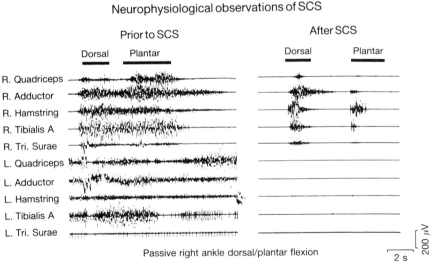

Neurophysiological observations of SCS

Figure 4.1. This shows the effect of spinal cord stimulation on proprioceptive manœuvres: passive stretch. These are surface EMG recordings during passive flexion and extension of the ankle as indicated by the horizontal bars. Passive dorsal and plantar flexion of the ankle elicits tonic proprioceptive reflexes. In spastic patients this typically results in excessive EMG activity, which may extend to the contralateral limb as indicated on the left. Spinal cord stimulation reduces such activity and completely suppresses spread of reflexes to the contralateral leg (from Dimitrijević *et al.* 1986).

Spinal cord stimulation is a technique of producing afferent stimulation in order to modify abnormal motor control in patients with upper motor neuron disorders, and is presumably mediated via dorsal columns, the autonomic nervous system, and the propriospinal interneuron system. In patients with excessive spasticity, coactivation of muscles occurs, with a resulting decrease in motor function. An improvement in motor function following reduction of spasticity in multiple sclerosis and spinal cord injury patients has been demonstrated following spinal cord stimulation (Dimitrijević *et al.* 1978, 1980; Read *et al.* 1980; Siegfried *et al.* 1981; Illis *et al.* 1980; Dimitrijević *et al.* 1986*a*,*b*). Figure 4.1 indicates the kind of responses which may be seen with spinal cord stimulation in patients with spinal cord injury, and indicates that after a period of spinal cord stimulation, voluntary activity tends to be more controlled, with less inadvertent coactivation of inappropriate muscle groups. Possibly repetitive stimulation via spinal cord stimulation activates dorsal columns and related brainstem structures, which in turn modify descending motor volleys and thus influence segmental reflexes (see Sherwood 1985).

References

Bajd, T., Gregoric, M., Vodovnik, L. and Benko, H. (1985). Electrical stimulation in treating spasticity due to spinal cord injury. *Archives of Physical Medicine*, **66**, 515–17.

Brausch, U., Henatsch, H. D., Student, C., and Takano, K. (1973). The effect of diazepam on development of stretch reflex tension. In *The benzodiazepines* (ed. S. Garattini, E. Mussini, and L. O. Randall), pp. 531–43. Raven Press, New York.

Brodal, A. (1969). *Neurological anatomy*, pp. 151–255. Oxford University Press, London.

Cook, J. B. and Nathan P. W. (1967). On the site of action of diazepam in spasticity in man. *Journal of Neurological Science*, **5**, 33–7.

Corcos, D. M., Gottlieb, G. L., Penn, R. D., Myklebust, B., and Agarwal, G. C. (1986). Movement deficits caused by hyperexcitable stretch reflexes in spastic humans. *Brain*, **109**, 1043–58.

Dhawan, B. N. and Sharma, J. N. (1970). Facilitation of the flexor reflex in the cat by the intrathecal injection of catecholamines. *British Journal of Pharmacology*, **40**, 237–48.

Dimitrijević, M. R. and Nathan, P. W. (1967). Studies of spasticity in man: I: Some features of spasticity. *Brain*, **90**, 1–30.

Dimitrijević, M. R., Sherwood, A. M., and Nathan, P. W. (1978). Clonus: peripheral and central mechanisms. In *Progress in Clinical Neurophysiology*, Vol. 9 (ed. J. E. Desmedt), pp. 173–82. Karger, Basle.

Dimitrijević, M. R., Nathan, P. W., and Sherwood, A. M. (1980). Clonus: The role of cental mechanisms, *Journal of Neurology, Neurosurgery and Psychiatry*, **43**, 321–32.

Dimitrijević, M. M., Dimitrijević, M. R., Illis, L. S., Nakajima, K., Sharkey, P. C., and Sherwood, A. M. (1986*a*). Spinal cord stimulation for the control of spasticity in patients with chronic spinal cord injury. I. Clinical Observations. *C.N.S. Trauma*, **3**, 129–44.

Dimitrijević, M. R., Illis, L. S., Nakajima, K., Sharkey, P. C., and Sherwood, A. M. (1986*b*). Spinal cord stimulation for the control of spasticity in patients with chronic spinal cord injury. II: Neurophysiological Observations. *C.N.S. Trauma*, **3**, 145–52.

Dimitrijević, M. M., Dimitrijević, M. R., Verhagen-Metman, L., and Partridge, M. (1987). *Modification by muscle tone in patients with upper motor neuron dysfunctions by electrical stimulation of the sural nerve.* American Academy of Clinical Neurophysiology, Abstracts, Vol. 2, 9. The Academy, Boston, Mass.

Erickson, D. L., Blacklock, J. B., Michaelson, M., Sperling, K. B., and Lo, J. N. (1985). Control of spasticity by implantable continuous flow morphine pump. *Neurosurgery*, **16**, 215–17.

Foerster, O. (1911). Restriction of the posterior nerve roots of the spinal cord. *Lancet*, **2**, 76–9.

Foerster, O. (1936). Motorische felder und bahnen. In *Handbuch der Neurologie* (ed. O. Bumke and O. Foerster), **6**, 1–357.

Herman, R. M., Wainberg, M. D., Delguidice, P. F., and Willscher, M. K. (1988). The effect of low dose intrathecal morphine on impaired micturition reflexes in human subjects with spinal cord lesions *Anesthesiology*, **69**, 313–18.

Illis, L. S. (1963). Changes in spinal cord synapses and a possible explanation for spinal shock. *Experimental Neurology*, **8**, 328–35.

Illis, L. S. (1967). The relative densities of monosynaptic pathways to cells and dendrites in the ventral horn. *Journal of Neurological Science*, **4**, 259–70.

Illis, L. S. (1973). An experimental model of regeneration in the CNS. I: Synaptic changes. *Brain*, **96**, 47–60.

Illis, L. S. (1988). Clinical evaluation and pathophysiology of the spinal cord in the chronic stage. In *Spinal cord dysfunction: assessment* (ed. L. S. Illis), pp. 107–28. Oxford University Press.

Illis, L. S., Sedgwick, E. M., and Tallis, R. (1980). Spinal cord stimulation in multiple sclerosis: clinical results. *Journal of Neurology, Neurosurgery and Psychiatry*, **43**, 1–14.

Jones, R. F. (1971). Lioresal in the control of spasticity. In *Spasticity—a topical survey* (ed. W. Birkmeyer), pp. 110–112. Hans Huber, Vienna.

Kato, M., Waldmann, U., and Murakami, S. (1978). Effects of baclofen on spinal neurones of cats. *Neuropharmacology*, **17**, 827–33.

McLellan, D. L. (1973). Effect of baclofen upon monosynaptic and tonic vibration reflexes in patients with spasticity. *Journal of Neurology, Neurosurgery and Psychiatry*, **36**, 555–60.

McLellan, D. L. (1977). Co-contraction and stretch reflexes in spasticity during treatment with baclofen. *Journal of Neurology, Neurosurgery and Psychiatry*, **40**, 30–8.

Melzack, R. and Wall, P. D. (1965). Pain mechanisms: a new theory. *Science*, **150**, 971–9.

Michaelis, L. S. (1976). Spasticity in spinal cord injuries. In *Handbook of clinical neurology* (ed. P. J. Vinken and G. W. Bruyn), pp. 477–87 (Chapter 26). North-Holland, Amsterdam.

Nathan, P. W. (1959). Intrathecal phenol to relieve spasticity in paraplegia. *Lancet*, **2**, 1099–1102.

Nathan, P. W. (1965). Relief of spasticity. *British Medical Journal*, **1**, 1096–1100.

Penn, R. D. and Kroin, J. S. (1987). Long-term intrathecal baclofen infusion for treat-ment of spasticity. *Journal of Neurosurgery*, **66**, 181–5.

Pierrot-Deseilligny, E. (1983). Pathophysiology of spasticity. *Triangle*, **22**, 165–74.

Pineli, P. (1973). Electromyographic evaluation of drug-induced muscle relaxation. In *The benzodiazepines* (ed. S. Garattini, E. Mussini, and L. O. Randall), pp. 559–64. Raven Press, New York.

Przybyla, A. C. and Wang, S. C. (1968). Locus of central depressant action of diazepam. *Journal of Pharmacological and Experimental Therapy*, **163**, 439–47.

Read, D. J., Matthews, W. D. and Higson, R. H. (1980). The effect of spinal cord stimulation on patients with multiple sclerosis. *Brain*, **103**, 803–33.

Roby, A., Bussel, B., and Willer, J. C. (1981). Morphine reinforces post-discharge inhibition of alpha motoneurones in Man. *Brain Research*, **222**, 209–12.

Sachais, B. A., Logue, J. N., and Carey, M. S. (1977). Baclofen: a new antispastic drug. *Archives of Neurology (Chicago)*, **34**, 422–8.

Scheibel, M. E. and Scheibel, A. B. (1966). Spinal motorneurons, interneurons and Renshaw cells. *Archives of Italian Biology*, **104**, 328–53.

Sherwood, A. M. (1985). Electrical stimulation of the spinal cord in movement dis-orders. In *Neural stimulation* (ed. J. B. Myklebust, J. F. Cusick, A. Sances, and S. J. Larson), pp. 111–46. CRC Press, Boca Raton, Florida.

Siegfried, J., Lazoerthes, Y., and Broggi, G. (1981). Electrical SCS for spastic move-ment disorders. *Applied Neurophysiology*, **44**, 77–92.

Stratten, W. and Barnes, C. D. (1971). Diazepam and presynaptic inhibition. *Neuro-pharmacology*, **10**, 685–96.

Struppler, A. (1985). Some new aspects of spasticity. In *Clinical neurophysiology in spasticity* (ed. P. J. Delwaide and R. R. Young), pp. 95–107. Elsevier, Amsterdam.

Wainberg, M. C., Herman, R. M., Willscher M. K., and Delguidice, P. F. (1987). The effect of low-dose intrathecal morphine on bladder capacity in human subjects with spinal cord lesions. *Society for Neuroscience Abstracts*, **13**, 1302.

Willer, J. C. and Bussel, B. (1980). Evidence for a direct spinal mechanism in morphine-induced inhibition of nociceptive reflexes in humans. *Brain Research*, **187**, 212–15.

5

Spasticity II: Physiological measurements

E. M. Sedgwick and J. Benfield

The gamma motor system

The most attractive animal model of spasticity has been the decerebrate cat, whose rigidity has been shown to depend on active gamma-motor-neurons which give a high gain to the stretch reflex by activating the muscle spindles: the gamma loop hypothesis.

Direct tests by microneuronographic recording of muscle afferent fibres of spastic human subjects show that the gamma system is not overactive, and the muscle spindles do not have an increased sensitivity to stretch in spasticity. These are technically difficult experiments, during which the subject must be lying at rest, and rather few subjects have been tested; but the role of an over-active gamma system can be excluded at least for the conditions under which these experiments were undertaken (Burke 1983).

A substantial body of work has compared the human H reflex with the tendon (T) reflex in an attempt to separate the contributions of the mono-synaptic reflex as against those of the gamma system. The rationale was that both electrical stimulation of the tibial nerve and a tap of the tendo Achilles would produce a monosynaptic reflex contraction of the soleus. The electrical stimulus, however, would bypass the muscle spindle, and produce an H reflex of amplitude dependent only upon the excitability of the mono-synaptic reflex. A tendon tap would excite a larger or smaller muscle afferent volley depending on whether or not the muscle spindles were sensitized by gamma motor-fibre activity. Comparison of the H and T reflexes would then indicate the activity in the gamma system. The underlying assumptions are that the tendon tap and electrical stimulus are equivalent and synchronous stimuli; unfortunately they are not. A tendon tap produces a wave of vibration spreading through the muscle, and muscles' spindles are excited asynchronously, producing an input volley to the spinal cord lasting as long as 20–30 msec. This allows time for polysynaptic segmental effects on motor neurons as well as the known monosynaptic reflex, and the resultant twitch is likely to be a product of both (Burke *et al.* 1984).

The alpha-motor-neuron

Another hypothesis has been that spasticity is the result of increased excitability of the alpha-motor-neuron to input from the muscle spindles. Two techniques have been used to study this, and the outcome is reasonably clear within the limitations of the original hypothesis.

The H reflex is the best test of the monosynaptic reflex excitability. As the stimulus to the tibial nerve is increased, the H response of the soleus muscle increases to a maximum and then decreases due to the contaminating effects of direct excitation of motor fibres. This makes up the recruitment curve of the H reflex. The curves of normal and spastic subjects look qualitatively similar (direct numerical comparisons between subjects are not possible for methodological reasons). Measurement of the maximum H reflex (H_{max}) and maximum motor response (M_{max}) when all the motor efferents are directly stimulated gives an estimate of the proportion of the motor neuron pool responsive to a muscle spindle input. The results from several laboratories tend to support the hypothesis that more motor neurons are excited by a Ia volley in spastics, but the results are far from convincing. There is a wide variation in both normals and spastics (Burke 1988).

Table 5.1. Summary of the changes in spinal segmental inhibitory mechanisms in patients after spinal injury.

Inhibition	Spinal injury
Ia Reciprocal inhibition	Enhanced
Ib Golgi inhibition	? No reports
Vibration TVR Vibration inhibition of H-reflex	TVR becomes phasic
D1- presynaptic	Enhanced
Renshaw inhibition	Present but variable

A more indirect look at motor neuron response to muscle spindle input can be achieved by vibrating a muscle which produces a vibration reflex. The reflex involves several segmental and suprasegmental mechanisms, so indirect inference about the excitability of the motor neurons can be drawn. In normal subjects the reflex is sustained and tonic: in spinal spasticity vibration produces a poor sustained phasic response (Dimitrijević *et al.* 1977).

Lack of inhibition

Spasticity is often explained as being the result of a loss of inhibition. In fact the long descending pathways are all excitatory in action; they may terminate on segmental inhibitory neurons, but they themselves are excitatory. It is possible to study some of the segmental inhibitory mechanisms in man. The techniques depend on the H reflex and changes in it following conditioning stimuli of appropriate strength to the same (tibial) or other nerves. Figure 5.1 shows the segmental inhibitory pathways that have been extensively studied in animals (Lundberg 1975).

Renshaw inhibition

Motor neuron axon collaterals excite Renshaw cells, which, in turn, inhibit motor neurons of the same pool. The role of this inhibitory mechanism in the control of movement is not fully understood, and absence of Renshaw

Spinal segmental inhibitory mechanisms

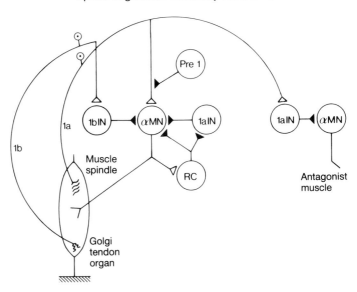

Fig. 5.1. The major spinal segmental inhibitory neurons are shown diagrammatically. Ia and Ib are afferent fibres from muscle spindles and Golgi tendon organs respectively; αMN, alpha-motor-neuron; IaIN, inhibitory interneuron on to which a branch of the Ia afferent fibre projects; RC, Renshaw cell innervated by recurrent collateral from the alpha-motor-neuron; IbIN, interneuron on to which the Golgi tendon afferent projects; PreI, interneurons involved in presynaptic inhibition. All the neurons except the motor neurons are inhibitory.

inhibition would not be expected to lead to spasticity. The Renshaw cell axons, however, also project to, and can inhibit, the Ia inhibitory interneuron.

Measurement of Renshaw inhibition in man is difficult and involved, and could not be achieved in one-third of subjects (Hultborn *et al.* 1979). Normal subjects showed greater Renshaw inhibition during gentle contraction of the soleus muscle, and relatively less when the muscle was contracted more forcefully. In a large series of subjects with spastic haemiplegia, one-third gave no result (the same proportion as in normals), 13 per cent showed more inhibition than normals, and the remainder were similar to the control group. Far from showing a lack of inhibition, these results showed normal or increased inhibition in spastic haemiplegia (Katz and Pierrot-Deseilligny 1982).

Reciprocal Ia inhibition

Reciprocal inhibition of antagonistic muscle groups around a joint has been extensively researched in the cat and monkey spinal cord (see Lundberg 1975; Baldissera *et al.* 1981). There is a disynaptic linkage between Ia afferents and antagonist alpha-motor-neurons via a single inhibitory Ia inter-neuron. Furthermore there is a marked similarity between descending and segmental input to the agonist motor neuron and inhibitory interneuron, suggesting they can be used in parallel to co-ordinate movement around a joint.

Reciprocal inhibition in ankle extensors in man was studied by Mizuno *et al.* (1971). Stimulation of low-threshold afferents, which include muscle spindle afferents, in the common peroneal nerve resulted in short latency (1–2 msec) inhibition of the ipsilateral soleus H-reflex. Using single conditioning pulses of strength close to the motor threshold for peroneal nerve motor axons, no effect was found in normal subjects ($n=7$) at rest, but inhibition of the H reflex by 35–100 per cent was clearly seen in four of six patients with bilateral athetosis of cerebral palsy, technical problems preventing measurements in the other two. Tanaka (1974) confirmed the absence of reciprocal inhibition in normal subjects at rest and its presence during voluntary dorsi-flexion.

Recent work has produced a rather different picture. Crone *et al.* (1985) could not confirm the Japanese findings (Tanaka 1974; Shindo *et al.* 1984). Further studies on sixty normal subjects (Crone *et al.* 1987) revealed a mean inhibition of soleus H-reflex at rest of 14.9 per cent: much more than previously described.

H-reflexes are not normally found at rest in tibialis anterior, although Teasdall *et al.* (1952) reported them in patients with lower brainstem or upper cervical lesions. It was suggested that ankle dorsiflexor motor neurons are tonically suppressed at rest, possibly as a result of descending tonic excitation in ankle extensor motor neurons, and hence in their Ia inhibitory interneurons, which project on to tibialis anterior motor neurons.

Active dorsiflexion at the ankle inhibits the soleus H-reflex. In common with that of the cat, the extensor motor neuron pool in man seems to be kept tonically more excitable than the flexor pool. This is presumably due to descending vestibular influences.

The idea of descending and segmental inputs both driving the Ia inhibitory interneuron came from work by Simoyama and Tanaka (1973), which showed that Ia inhibition to soleus MN during dorsiflexion began prior to the onset of EMG changes in the pretibial muscles. This descending drive to the Ia interneuron must be reduced or abolished as a result of spinal injury, and would result in a reduction of Ia inhibition. It is not clear whether descending control operates via excitation of inhibitory interneurons or by decreased presynaptic inhibition of Ia afferents. A decrease in presynaptic inhibition of Ia fibres on soleus motor neurons at the onset of plantar flexion has recently been demonstrated in man (Hultborn et al. 1987). In a study of the discharge probability patterns of human motor neurons in health and in spinal spasticity, it was found that transmission in the reciprocal inhibitory pathway was enhanced. These ideas need further testing in man, but there seems to be no loss of reciprocal inhibition (Ashby and Wiens 1989).

D1 inhibition

Conditioning stimuli to the peroneal nerve can inhibit the soleus H reflex at condition-test intervals of 0–5 msec, and this has already been shown to be a manifestation of the Ia reciprocal inhibitory mechanism. If the condition–test interval is prolonged beyond 5 msec, and if the conditioning stimulus to the peroneal nerve is increased to become a volley of 2–5 pulses at 1.5 times the motor threshold, then a second period of inhibition can be observed, lasting 5–80 msec. This is called D1 (Depression 1) and possibly reflects a pre-synaptic mechanism (Tanaka 1974). El-Tohamy and Sedgwick (1983) produced circumstantial evidence that group II muscle afferents were the effective afferent fibres.

In spinal man, D1 is present even in subjects still in spinal shock (Carter et al. 1987; Benfield et al. 1988). In many patients the degree of inhibition, 50 per cent in normal subjects, was increased to 80–90 per cent at its maximum, but the time course was shorter. Even patients studied during spinal shock and who had enhanced D1 inhibition subsequently became spastic and still had enhanced D1.

In a small group of patients with spastic haemiplegia, no D1 inhibition was found on the affected side. One cannot assume that the same neurophysio-logical disorder underlies both haemiplegic and paraplegic spasticity (El Tohamy and Sedgwick 1982).

Summary

Knowledge gained from study of spinal segmental mechanisms in animals has allowed hypotheses about the nature of human spasticity to be tested. So far the hypotheses involving change in excitability of the gamma motor system and loss of inhibition have been found wanting. The results are summarized in Table 5.1.

New methodologies are developing, such as magnetic stimulation and magnetic recording, which will allow testing of other hypotheses. When a satisfactory physiological explanation of spasticity is available then our efforts at treatment and management can be more logically directed.

References

Ashby, P. and Wiens, M. (1989). Reciprocal inhibition following lesions of the spinal cord in man. *Journal of Physiology*, **414**, 145–57.

Baldissera, F., Hultborn, H., and Illert, M. (1981). Integration of spinal neuronal systems. In *Handbook of physiology*, Section I, *The nervous system*, Vol. 2, *Motor control* (ed. V. B. Brooks), pp. 509–95. American Physiological Society, Bethesda, Maryland.

Benfield, J., Russell, J., and Sedgwick, E. M. (1988). The H reflex and D1 inhibition during spinal shock in man. *Journal of Physiology*, **406**, 155P.

Burke, D. (1983). Critical examination of the case for or against fusimotor involvement in disorders of muscle tone. In *Motor control mechanisms in health and disease*, Advances in Neurology, Vol. 39 (ed. J. E. Desmedt), pp. 133–50. Raven Press, New York.

Burke, D., Gandevia, S. C., and McKeon, B. (1984). Monosynaptic and oligosynaptic contributions to human ankle jerk and H reflex. *Journal of Neurophysiology*, **52**, 435–48.

Burke, D. (1988). Spasticity as an adaptation to pyramidal tract injury. In *Functional recovery in neurological disease*, Advances in Neurology, Vol. 47 (ed. S. G. Waxman). Raven Press, New York.

Carter, M. R., Rowe, I. C. M., and Sedgwick, E. M. (1988). D1 inhibition in man with spinal cord injury. *Journal of Physiology*, **396**, 157P.

Crone, C., Hultborn, H., and Jespersen, B. (1985). Reciprocal inhibition from the peroneal nerve to soleus motorneurones with special reference to the size of the H reflex. *Experimental Brain Research*, **59**, 418–22.

Crone, C., Hultborn, H., and Jespersen, B. (1987). Reciprocal Ia inhibition between ankle flexors and extensors in man. *Journal of Physiology*, **389**, 163–85.

Dimitrijević, M. R., Spencer, W., Trontelj, J., and Dimitrijević, M. (1977). Reflex effects of vibration in patients with spinal cord lesions. *Neurology*, **27**, 1078–86.

El-Tohamy and Sedgwick, E. M. (1982). Spinal inhibitory mechanisms in spasticity. *Electroencephalography and clinical neurophysiology*, **53**, 3P.

El-Tohamy and Sedgwick, E. M. (1983). Spinal inhibition in man: depression of soleus H reflex by stimulation of the nerve to the antagonist muscle. *Journal of Physiology*, **336**, 497–508.

Hultborn, H. and Pierrot-Deseilligny, E. (1979). Changes in recurrent inhibition during voluntary soleus contractions in man studied by an H-reflex method. *Journal of Physiology*, **292**, 229–52.

Hultborn, H., Meunier, S., Morin, C., and Pierrot-Deseilligny, E. (1987). Changes in presynaptic inhibition of Ia fibres at the onset of voluntary contraction in man. *Journal of Physiology*, **389**, 757–72.

Katz, R. and Pierrot-Deseilligny, E. (1982). Recurrent inhibition of alpha motorneurons in patients with upper motor neuron lesions. *Brain*, **105**, 103–24.

Lundberg, A. (1975). Control of spinal mechanisms from the brain. In *The nervous system*, Vol. 1 (ed. D. B. Tower). New York, Raven Press.

Mizuno, Y., Tanaka, R., and Yanagisawa, N. (1971). Reciprocal group I inhibition on triceps surae motorneurons in man. *Journal of Neurophysiology*, **34**, 1010–17.

Shindo, M., Harayama, H., Kondo, K., Yanagisawa, N., and Tanaka, R. (1984). Changes in reciprocal inhibition during voluntary contractions in man. *Experimental Brain Research*, **53**, 400–8.

Shimoyama, M. and Tanaka, R. (1973). Reciprocal inhibition at the onset of voluntary contraction in man. *Journal of the Physiological Society of Japan*, **35**, 513–14.

Tanaka, R. (1974). Reciprocal Ia inhibition and voluntary movements in man. *Experimental Brain Research*, **21**, 529–40.

Teasdall, R. D., Park, A. M., Langruth, H. W., and Magladery, J. W. (1952). Electrophysiological studies of reflex activity in patients with lesions of the nervous system. II: Disclosure of normally suppressed monosynaptic reflex discharge of spinal motorneurones by lesions of lower brain-stem and spinal cord. *Bulletin of the Johns Hopkins Hospital*, **91**, 245–56.

Yanagisawa, N., Tanaka, R., and Ito, Z. (1976). Reciprocal inhibition in spastic hemiplegia of man. *Brain*, **99**, 555–74.

6

Management of cardio-vascular abnormalities caused by autonomic dysfunction in spinal cord injury

C. J. Mathias, H. L. Frankel, and J. D. Cole

Introduction

The activity of the autonomic nervous system is dependent on a cranial parasympathetic outflow and on spinal pathways, which traverse the cervical, thoracic, and lumbar sections of the spinal cord, with the sympathetic outflow emerging from the thoracic and upper lumbar segments, and the parasympathetic outflow from the sacral segments. In patients with spinal cord lesions the major proportion of the autonomic outflow may therefore be disrupted, resulting in inactivity, or dissociation of actions from cerebral regulation. A greater degree of disordered cardio-vascular control often occurs in patients with cervical and high thoracic spinal cord lesions. Activity of the autonomic nervous system, however, is also dependent on the afferent nervous system (Fig. 6.1), and the level and extent of lesion thus influences responses. This review will concentrate on the management of cardio-vascular abnormalities which result from autonomic dysfunction in patients with high spinal cord injury. The initial description will be in patients with acute lesions (in spinal shock, when they have substantial impairment of even isolated spinal cord function), as their cardio-vascular problems are often different from those in the chronic stages. The pathophysiological basis of autonomic disorders in spinal cord injuries has been described in detail previously (Frankel and Mathias 1976; Mathias and Frankel 1983a, 1988; Cole 1988).

Recent spinal cord injury

In the early stages the basal systolic and diastolic blood-pressures in high spinal cord lesions are usually lower than normal even in the horizontal position, in which the majority are nursed (Walsh 1960; Meinecke et al. 1971). This reflects absent tonic brainstem sympathetic vasoconstrictor impulses and an overall reduction in sympathetic nervous activity, which is reflected in low plasma noradrenalin and adrenalin levels (Mathias et al.

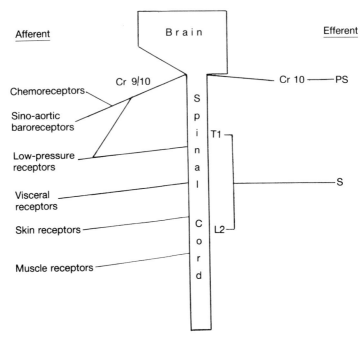

Fig. 6.1. Schematic outline of the major autonomic pathways controlling the circulation. The major afferent input into the central nervous system is through the glossopharyngeal (Cr, 9) and vagus (Cr, 10) nerves by activation of baroreceptors in the carotid sinus and aortic arch. Chemoreceptors and low-pressure receptors also influence the efferent outflow. The latter consists of the cranial parasympathetic (PS) outflow to the heart via the vagus nerves, and the sympathetic outflow from the thoracic and upper lumbar segments of the spinal cord. Activation of visceral, skin, and muscle receptors, in addition to cerebral stimulation, influences the efferent outflow (from Mathias and Frankel 1988).

1979*a*) (Fig. 6.2). Peripheral vasodilatation may predispose to increased vascular permeability, subcutaneous oedema, and skin breakdown, which is common in the early stages of spinal injuries. Low blood-pressure does not, as a rule, warrant corrective measures; but the absence of intact baroreflex pathways renders such patients susceptible to hypotension in situations where a compensatory increase in sympathetic activity is needed; reduction in intravascular volume, and even a minor degree of bleeding or dehydration, may thus lower blood-pressure substantially, as do manœuvres such as even a minor degree of head-up tilt. The reverse, an excessive elevation in blood-pressure, may occur if intravascular volume is expanded because of a rapid infusion of blood or intravenous fluids.

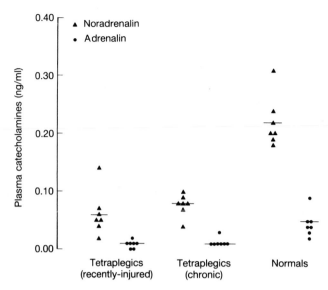

Fig. 6.2. Resting levels of plasma noradrenalin and adrenalin in recently injured tetraplegics in spinal shock, in chronically injured tetraplegics, and in normal age-matched subjects. The horizonal bar indicates the mean value. Basal plasma catechol-amine levels in both recently injured and chronically injured tetraplegics are about 35 per cent of normal levels (from Mathias *et al.* 1979*a*).

In contrast to patients with chronic spinal cord injuries (in whom there is recovery of isolated spinal cord function), a variety of stimuli below the lesion (such as cutaneous cold, pain, or urinary bladder or large bowel distension), do not elevate blood-pressure; with isolated spinal cord recovery, however, this changes, and the cardio-vascular disturbances which form part of the syndrome of autonomic dysreflexia often ensue (Mathias 1976*a*; Mathias *et al.* 1979*a*) (Fig. 6.3). The lack of response to such stimuli in the early stages reflects the inability to activate spinally dependent sympathetic reflexes. There is no evidence of diminished vascular respons-iveness, as patients in the acute phase also have an enhanced response to pressor agents such as noradrenalin, as do chronically injured tetraplegics (Fig. 6.4).

The basal heart-rate is often on the low side, partially because of a sympathetic/parasympathetic imbalance resulting in relative overactivity of the cardiac vagus. Changes in heart-rate are clinically important, and a persistent bradycardia may provide a vital clue to hypothermia, which may be missed if only oral temperature is recorded (Pledger 1962) (Fig. 6.5). In the early stages such patients are particularly prone to hypothermia, as they are unable to shiver. This major mechanism for thermogenesis, in addition to

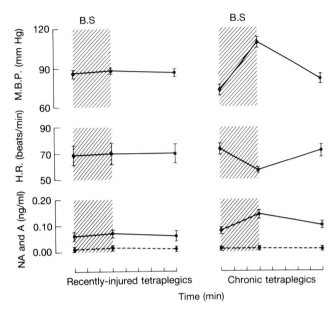

Fig. 6.3. Average levels of mean blood-pressure (MBP), heart-rate (HR), and plasma noradrenalin levels (NA, continuous line) and adrenalin (A, interrupted line) in recently injured and chronically injured tetraplegics, before, during, and after bladder stimulation (BS). The bars indicate SEM ±. No changes occurred in recently injured tetraplegics, unlike the chronic tetraplegics, in whom MBP and plasma NA levels rise, and HR fails. There are no changes in plasma A levels in either group (from Mathias *et al.* 1979*a*).

the absence of vasoconstriction and thus an inappropriate peripheral vasodilatation, may lower temperature substantially. The monitoring of temperature (with a low-reading rectal thermometer), and also heart-rate are useful guides, as the inability to vasoconstrict peripherally further enhances the likelihood of hypothermia and increases the difficulties of its detection in such patients.

A problem of major importance may occur in patients with high cervical cord lesions which also involve the C4/5 segments supplying the phrenic nerves, as they are dependent on artificial respiration. Tracheal suction and toilet is needed at regular intervals, and bradycardia and cardiac arrest may readily occur, especially in patients who are hypoxic (Dolphus and Frankel 1965; Frankel *et al.* 1975; Mathias *et al.* 1976*b*). The reasons for this response are provided in Table 6.1 and Fig. 6.6. Overactivity of the cardiac vagi can be readily prevented by blocking peripheral muscarinic receptors with atropine. Bradycardia and cardiac arrest may also occur in chronic

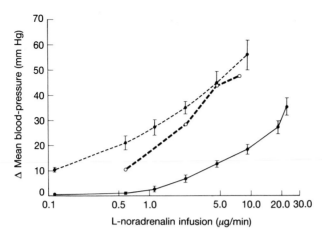

Fig. 6.4. Changes (Δ) in average mean blood-pressure during different dose infusion-rates of noradrenalin given intravenously to 5 chronic tetraplegics (filled circles, interrupted line), 3 recently injured tetraplegics (open circles, interrupted lines), and 10 control subjects (filled circles, continuous line). The bars indicate SEM ±. There is an enhanced pressor response to noradrenalin in both groups of tetraplegics over the dose-range studied (from Mathias *et al.* 1976*b* and 1979*a*).

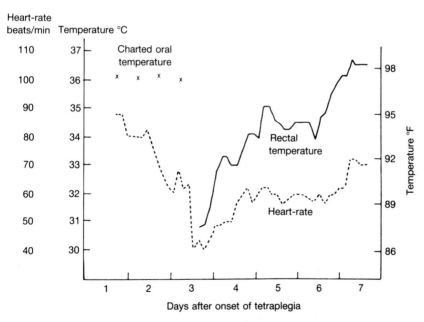

Fig. 6.5. Fall in core temperature (measured as rectal temperature) and in heart-rate in a recently injured tetraplegic in a temperate climate. Hypothermia is best monitored with a low reading rectal thermometer, and, as indicated, may be missed if oral temperature only is recorded (from Pledger 1962).

Table 6.1. The major mechanisms contributing to bradycardia and cardiac arrest in recently injured tetraplegics in spinal shock. Some of the management approaches are indicated.

	Tracheal suction	Hypoxia
Normal:	Increased sympathetic nervous activity causes tachycardia and raises blood-pressure	Bradycardia is the primary response, opposed by the pulmonary (inflation) vagal reflex, resulting in tachycardia.
Tetraplegics:	No increase in sympathetic nervous activity, therefore no rise in heart-rate or blood-pressure. Vagal afferent stimulation may lead to unopposed vagal efferent activity.	Bradycardia, the primary response, is not opposed by the pulmonary (inflation) vagal reflex (because of disconnection from respirator or fixed respiration).
	Increased vagal cardiac tone (bradycardia and cardiac arrest)	
Management:	Oxygen Reconnection to Atropine Isoprenaline Demand pacemaker respirator	

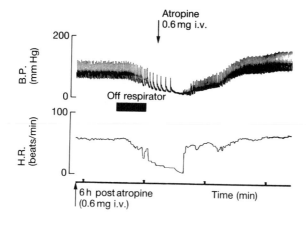

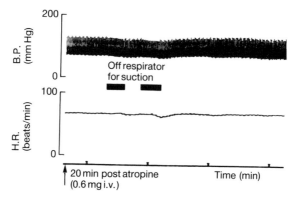

Fig. 6.6. Blood-pressure (BP) and heart-rate (HR) in a recently injured tetraplegic (C4/5 lesion) in spinal shock, 6 hours after the last dose of intravenous atropine (upper panel). Disconnecting the respirator, as required for aspirating the airways, resulted in sinus bradycardia and cardiac arrest (which was also observed on the electrocardiograph). This was reversed by reconnection, intravenous atropine, and external cardiac message. The lower panel shows the effect of disconnection from the respirator and tracheal suction 20 minutes after atropine, which now prevents the changes in heart-rate and also blood-pressure (from Frankel *et al.* 1975 and Mathias 1976*b*).

tetraplegics, for example during endotracheal intubation following administration of muscle relaxants (Welply *et al.* 1975) (Fig. 6.7). The vagovaal reflex causing cardiac arrest appears similar to the responses described in recently injured tetraplegics, and can be prevented by intravenous atropine prior to intubation.

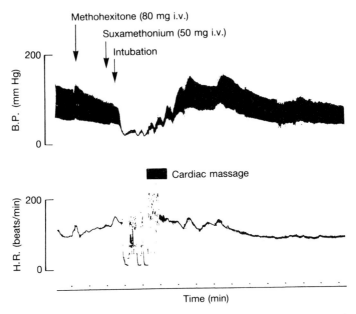

Fig. 6.7. The effect of endotracheal intubation on blood-pressure (BP) and heart-rate (HR) in a chronically injured tetraplegic being anaesthetized for urological surgery. Because of the delay in the operation list, the effects of atropine in the premedication had presumably worn off. Intubation was followed by cardiac arrest, which was reversed by oxygen and external cardiac message (from Welply *et al.* 1975).

Chronic spinal cord injury

In such patients isolated spinal cord function has recovered, and cardio-vascular disorders result from both dissociation of cerebral regulation and abnormal reflexes functioning at a spinal level. The autonomic abnormalities also influence cardio-vascular responses to a variety of vasoactive agents. The disturbances are described below.

Postural hypotension

This is common in the early stages after spinal cord injury, and is especially noticeable during the early period of rehabilitation (Fig. 6.8a). Although prolonged inactivity may contribute, a major reason for the fall in blood-pressure during head-up change is the impairment of baroreceptor reflexes following transection of descending sympathetic vasoconstrictor pathways. A variety of manifestations suggestive of cerebral ischaemia may occur, and in some may culminate in syncope (Table 6.2). The symptoms diminish with

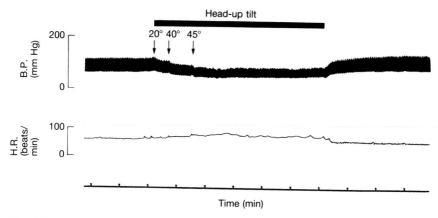

Fig. 6.8a. Blood-pressure (BP) and heart-rate (HR) in a tetraplegic patient before and after head-up tilt, in the early stages of rehabilitation, where there were few muscle spasms and minimal autonomic dysreflexia (from Frankel and Mathias 1976).

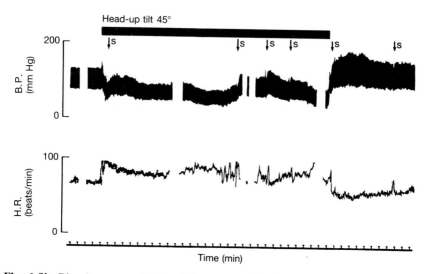

Fig. 6.8b. Blood-pressure (BP) and heart-rate (HR) in a tetraplegic patient before during and after head-up tilt to 45 per cent. Blood-pressure promptly falls, but with partial recovery—which in this case is linked to skeletal muscle spasms (S) inducing spinal sympathetic activity. Some of the later oscillations may be due to the rise in plasma renin, which was measured where there are interruptions in the intra-arterial record. In the later phases of tilt, skeletal muscle spasms occur more frequently, and further elevate the blood-pressure. On return to the horizontal, blood-pressure rises rapidly above the previous basal level, and then slowly returns to the horizontal. Heart-rate usually moves in the opposite direction, except during muscle spasms, when there is a transient increase (from Mathias and Frankel 1988).

Table 6.2. Signs and symptoms of postural hypotension

Giddiness, buzzing, and ringing in ears
Blurring, greying out, loss of vision
Tingling in hands. Syncope.
Facial pallor.
Hypotension. Tachycardia. Occasionally bradycardia.
Venous pooling in lower limbs with cyanotic discoloration.

frequent tilt and greater mobility (Guttmann 1976), and the mechanisms accounting for this may be multiple. An improvement in cerebral auto-regulation may be a factor, as such patients can tolerate considerably lower cerebral perfusion pressures while maintaining intact cerebral blood-flow (Eidelman 1973). During head-up tilt, despite the absence of reflex sym-pathetic vasoconstriction, secondary but slowly reacting compensatory mechanisms operate, sometimes in an exaggerated manner (Mathias *et al.* 1975; 1980) (Fig. 6.9). Renin is released from the juxtaglomerular cells of the kidney, and results in formation of the powerful vasoconstrictor, angiotensin-II, which in addition to acting directly on blood-vessels, stimulates the adrenal cortex to release the mineralocorticoid hormone, aldosterone, and thus causes salt retention, and subsequently, water retention (Mathias *et al.* 1984) (Fig. 6.9). The combination of vascular effects and increase in intra-vascular volume may contribute to the improvement in blood-pressure seen after frequent episodes of tilt.

A reduction in extracellular fluid volume may account for the worsening of postural hypotension or its tolerance, when previously asymptomatic patients have been in bed for only a few days. Tetraplegics, like patients with idiopathic autonomic failure (Mathias *et al.* 1986) exhibit a recumbency-induced diuresis (Kooner *et al.* 1987); when prolonged this may reduce both intravascular and extracellular fluid volume, thus enhancing the propensity to postural hypotension. Unlike the case with patients with autonomic failure (who usually have a greater degree of postural hypotension), there is no natriuresis in tetraplegics, probably because their renin–angiotensin–aldosterone system is more responsive. The phenomenon described above may also account for why patients with high lesions are exquisitely sensitive to diuretic agents, which would act in a similar manner but in addition to water loss cause sodium depletion.

The management of postural hypotension utilizes our knowledge of patho-physiological changes and compensatory mechanisms which could be used to benefit (Mathias 1987). Frequent head-up tilt is usually the best means of reducing the postural fall and acquiring symptomatic tolerance to the low

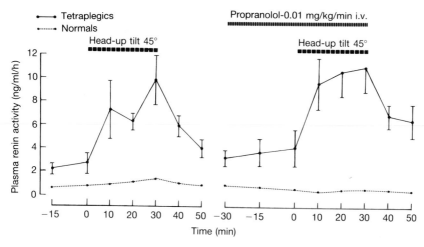

Fig. 6.9. Levels of plasma renin activity in tetraplegic patients (continuous lines) and in normal subjects (interrupted lines) before, during, and after head-up tilt to 45°. Levels in the left panel were before, and levels on the right after, administration of propranolol, in a dose which would have effectively blocked beta-adrenergic receptors. The renin response in the tetraplegics is considerably greater than in the normal subjects. Beta-blockade with propranolol had no effect on the renin response to head-up tilt in tetraplegics. This differs from the response in normal subjects. Taken in conjunction with other evidence, this suggests that renin release in tetraplegics during head-up tilt occurs independently of sympathetic activation and stimulation of beta-adrenergic receptors.

blood-pressure. Stimulation of spinal sympathetic reflexes through muscle spasms or visceral activity also helps to raise blood-pressure (Fig. 6.8b, p. 109). If necessary (and in particular in the early stages of rehabilitation), drugs (Table 6.3) are used. Ephedrine, 15 mg half an hour before changing posture is often effective; it acts both directly on blood-vessels and by enhancing release of noradrenalin from sympathetic nerve terminals. A variety of other agents which act through different mechanisms (Bannister and Mathias 1988) has been used. These include dihydroergotamine, indomethacin, and fludrocortisone; but such drugs are usually not necessary, as repeated head-up tilt offers the greatest benefit.

Autonomic dysreflexia

Stimulation of skin, viscera, or skeletal muscles below the level of the lesion results in a number of cardio-vascular (Fig. 6.10) and autonomic changes, which constitute the syndrome of autonomic dysreflexia (Guttmann and Whitteridge 1947) (Table 6.4). There is increased activity in many of the

Table 6.3. Some of the drugs used in reducing postural hypotension in autonomic failure patients and their site and mode of action. The drugs which have been used in tetraplegics and high spinal injuries are indicated by an asterisk

Vasoconstriction	
Resistance vessels	Ephedrine*
	Midodrine
Capacitance vessels	Dihydroergotamine*
Heart—stimulation	Xamoterol
Preventing vasodilatation	Indomethacin*
	Propranolol
Preventing nocturnal polyuria	Desmopressin (DDAVP)
Reducing salt-loss and plasma-volume expansion	Fludrocortisone

target organs supplied by the sympathetic and parasympathetic nervous system. The pathophysiological mechanisms responsible have been well described, and result from activation of afferent pathways (Table 6.5) in a variety of clinical situations, which via spinal reflexes result in an uncoordinated autonomic discharge—hence the term 'mass reflex'. The constriction of blood-vessels elevates blood-pressure, and may result in cold limbs (hence the term 'poikilothermia spinalis'); heart-rate often falls, because of increased vagal activity secondary to stimulation of the intact afferent limb of the baroreceptor reflex. The common stimuli causing autonomic dysreflexia are from the urinary bladder and the large bowel, with skeletal muscle spasms not infrequently contributing. The cardio-vascular changes are often short-lived, although a sustained level of hypertension may result, depending upon the persistence and the nature of the initiating stimulus. The paroxysmal nature of hypertension can occasionally cause concern about the possibility of phaeochromocytoma tumours, as patients often tend to vasodilate in the face and neck, have a throbbing headache, and sweat profusely in innervated areas of skin above the lesion. During autonomic dysreflexia, however, plasma noradrenalin levels rise from low basal levels (often 30 per cent of normal) to just above the normal range, indicative of sympathetic nervous activity as the cause of the changes (Mathias *et al.* 1976*a*). There is no change in plasma adrenalin, indicating

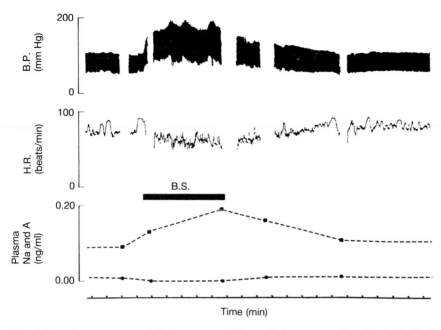

Fig. 6.10. Blood-pressure (BP), heart-rate (HR), and plasma noradrenalin (NA, filled squares) and adrenalin (A, filled circles) levels in a tetraplegic patient before, during, and after bladder stimulation (BS) induced by suprapubic percussion of the anterior abdominal wall. The rise in BP is initially accompanied by a rise in heart-rate, which then falls, as a result of increased vagal activity in response to the rise in pressure. Plasma NA, but not A, levels rise, suggesting an increase in sympathetic neural activity independently of adreno-medullary activation (from Mathias and Frankel 1986).

Table 6.4. Signs and symptoms of autonomic dys-reflexia

Pins and needles in innervated areas—neck, shoulders, arms

Fullness in head. Throbbing headache. Hot ears.

Tightness in chest, dyspnoea.

Elevation in blood-pressure. Fall in heart-rate.

Pupillary dilatation.

Pallor, initially followed by facial and cervical flushing, and sweating, in areas above and around the lesions.

Peripheral vasoconstriction. Cold hands and feet.

Table 6.5. Causes of autonomic dysreflexia

Cutaneous
  Pressure sores. Burns
  Infected toe-nails

Skeletal muscle
  Spasms, especially in limbs with contractures

Visceral
  Ureteric calculi
  Urinary bladder infection, distension by blocked catheter
    of discoordinated bladder, irritation by calculus,
    catheter, or bladder washout
  Anal fissures, faecal retention, or enemas
  Gastric ulceration or dilatation
  Cholecystitis or cholelithiasis
  Appendicitis
  Uterine contractions

Miscellaneous
  Ejaculatory procedures—intrathecal neostigmine or
    electro-ejaculation
  Vaginal dilatation
  Urethral catheter or abscess
  Bony fractures

---

that the changes are independent of adrenal medullary stimulation. The levels of both catecholamines are considerably lower than found in catecholamine-producing tumours.

Mild and transient episodes of autonomic dysreflexia occur frequently, and may be of value, especially when patients are sitting up, as they may reduce the posturally induced fall in blood-pressure. When prolonged, however, they may cause excessive sweating above the lesion, and a throbbing headache. Myocardial dysfunction and failure may occasionally occur. The greatest concern, however, relates to the neurological deficits which may result from either spasm of cerebral vessels or cerebral haemorrhage. These consist of epileptic seizures, visual deficits, and at times even extensive strokes or death.

The cornerstone in management of autonomic dysreflexia is determination of the site and nature of the initiating stimulus and alleviation of the precipitating cause. An anal fissure, for instance, may be difficult to demonstrate, especially in the absence of pain. To lower blood-pressure a variety of approaches may be used. If rapid lowering is needed head-up tilt, which causes venous pooling, may be useful. Drugs may be used, as indicated in Table 6.6. Many of these agents have the potential to lower blood-pressure

Table 6.6. Drugs used in the management of autonomic dys-reflexia, classified according to their major site of action

Afferent		Topical lignocaine
Spinal cord		Clonidine
		Reserpine
		Spinal anaesthetics
Efferent	Ganglia	Hexamethonium
	Nerve terminals	Guanethidine
	Alpha receptors	Phenoxybenzamine
Target organs	Blood-vessels	Glyceryl trinitrate
		Calcium channel blockers
	Sweat-glands	Probanthine

excessively, and this especially applies to drugs such as glyceryl trinitrate, which act directly on blood-vessels (Fig. 6.11). Clonidine does not usually lower blood-pressure below 'normal' basal levels, and, although it is reasonably successful in dampening hypertension (Mathias *et al.* 1979*b*), it may not be entirely effective in the low doses recommended, which avoid its known side-effects of sedation and dryness of mouth. Reserpine is one of the older antihypertensive agents, and may be of even greater benefit in resistant cases, as recent evidence indicates that it may prevent not only the actions of monoamine neurotransmitters released from sympathetic nerve endings, but also associated peptides, such as neuropeptide Y, which is a vasopressor agent in its own right, but is not affected by alpha-adrenoreceptor blockade (Lundberg *et al.* 1985).

Other approaches need to be considered in occasional patients, and these may include surgical procedures, such as rhizotomy and cordotomy or sacral and hypogastric neurotomy. These may be useful in patients with associated severe muscle spasms in whom drug therapy and/or alleviation of the cause is unsuccessful. Similar effects may also be achieved using non-surgical approaches, such as subarachnoid block with alcohol or phenol. The majority of these procedures, however, abolish spinal reflex activity, result in flaccid muscle paralysis and urinary bladder atony, and have disadvantages which need to be weighed against potential advantages. They should only be considered if all else has failed.

During surgery on the urinary tract, autonomic dysreflexia and hyper-tension can be a problem. If a general anaesthetic is used, increasing the

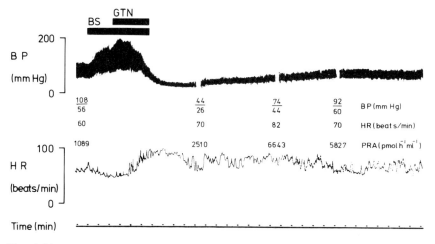

Fig. 6.11. Blood-pressure (BP) and heart-rate (HR) in a tetraplegic patient while supine, before, during, and after bladder stimulation (BS) induced by suprapubic percussion of the anterior abdominal wall. The elevation in blood-pressure is reversed by the administration of sublingual glyceryl trinitrate (GTN, 0.5 mg for $3\frac{1}{2}$ min), which rapidly reverses the hypertension, elevates the heart-rate, and then causes substantial hypotension. Levels of plasma renin activity (PRA) rise, presumably in response to the fall in blood-pressure (from Mathias and Frankel 1988).

concentration of halothane and raising intrathoracic pressure often success-fully controls the elevation in blood-pressure (Fig. 6.12) (Welply *et al.* 1975). Short-acting ganglionic blockers such as trimethaphan may be needed. Spinal anaesthesia, which suppresses the spinal component of the reflex arc, is often highly successful in preventing paroxysmal hypertension, and is also favoured in the management of hypertension and autonomic dysreflexia accompanying uterine contractions during delivery (Guttmann *et al.* 1965), as it usually avoids the need to proceed to a Caesarean section.

Sweating and headache are two other problems which cause much morbidity during autonomic dysreflexia (Schumacher and Guthrie 1951). Sweating can be excessive, and this can result in discomfort and in macera-tion of skin, thus enhancing the tendency to skin breakdown. Anticholinergic agents such as probanthine offer some benefit, and may be usefully combined with clonidine. The headache may be related to the level of hypertension, which when lowered will reduce the pain. It may however still remain; the use of aspirin and other simple analgesics such as paracetamol may provide benefit by acting on those mechanisms responsible for pain, which pre-sumably act in response to circulating or locally produced chemicals.

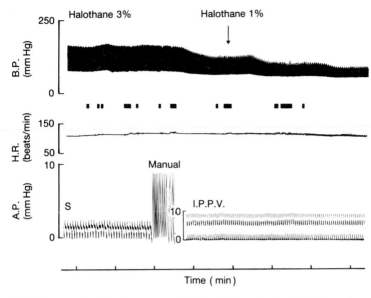

Fig. 6.12. Changes in blood-pressure (BP) and heart-rate (HR) in a chronically injured tetraplegic patient undergoing urological surgery. The dark blocks indicate where transurethral resection and diathermy was performed. Airway pressure (AP) is indicated when the patient was breathing spontaneously, was manually ventilated, and was on intermittent positive pressure ventilation (IPPV). The BP was initially satisfactorily controlled on 3 per cent halothane. Increasing airway pressure further reduces blood-pressure, and enables use of a lower concentration of halothane (1 per cent), which then successfully maintains the BP during resection and diathermy, which would otherwise elevate it considerably (from Welply *et al.* 1975).

Abnormal responses to vasoactive agents

The autonomic lesion predisposes patients with high spinal cord lesions to abnormal cardiovascular responses to vasoactive agents. This is of clinical importance, as there may be enhanced side-effects to the vasoactive properties of drugs which are not normally considered to cause cardio-vascular problems. This relates especially to the hypotensive actions of drugs which act directly on blood-vessels, such as glyceryl trinitrate. Vasodilators may be used beneficially to lower blood-pressure in an emergency; but one should be aware of their potential to induce severe hypotension.

An enhanced pressor response to the natural transmitter noradrenalin has long been recognized, the mechanisms responsible have been investigated, and the exaggerated responses are not exclusive to catecholamines but to a variety of pressor agents. A likely explanation appears to be the impairment of those autonomic reflexes which normally buffer a rise in blood-pressure; an increase in the population of various receptors on the target organs seems less likely, but cannot be excluded (Mathias *et al.* 1976*b*; Davies *et al.* 1982). Patients with high spinal lesions are 5–10 times more sensitive to the pressor effects of noradrenalin than normal subjects, and particular caution should be exercised when vasopressor agents are used in emergency situations.

The exaggerated responses to vasoactive agents, although for practical reasons less well studied, also occur in patients with early spinal cord injury, and the same degree of caution should therefore apply to this group.

Conclusion

Patients with high spinal cord lesions therefore manifest a number of cardio-vascular disorders which are directly linked to abnormalities of autonomic function. Their management and the therapeutic approaches used are dependent upon knowledge of the pathophysiological mechanisms involved; these encompass neural, hormonal, and biochemical derangements. The level of the lesion, its completeness, and the nature of the stimulus may singularly or together result in different responses, which can complicate the management; but the underlying principles described above are often a useful guideline in decisions on appropriate treatment.

References

Bannister, R. and Mathias, C. J. (1988). Management of postural hypotension. In Bannister, R., ed. *Autonomic failure: a textbook of clinical disorders of the autonomic nervous system* (2nd edn) (ed. R. Bannister), pp. 569–95. Oxford University Press.

Cole, J. D. (1988). The pathophysiology of the autonomic nervous system in spinal cord injury. In *Spinal cord dysfunction: assessment* (ed. L. S. Illis), pp. 201–35. Oxford University Press

Davies, I. B., Mathias, C. J., Sudera, D., and Sever, P. S. (1982). Agonist regulation of alpha-adrenergic receptor responses in man. *Journal of Cardiovascular Pharmacology*, **4**, S139–44.

Dolphus, P. and Frankel, H. L. (1965). Cardiovascular reflexes in tracheomatized tetraplegics. *Paraplegia*, **2**, 227.

Eidelman, B. H. (1973). Cerebral blood flow in normal and abnormal man. Unpublished D. Phil. thesis, University of Oxford.

Frankel, H. L. and Mathias, C. J. (1976). The cardiovascular system in paraplegia and tetraplegia. In *Handbook of clinical neurology*, Vol. 26, *Injuries of the spine and spinal cord*, Part II (ed. P. J. Vinken and G. W. Bruyn), Chapter 18, pp. 313–33. North-Holland Publishing Company, Amsterdam.

Frankel, H. L., Mathias, C. J., and Spalding, J. M. K. (1975). Mechanisms of reflex cardiac arrest in tetraplegic patients. *Lancet*, **ii**, 1183–5.

Guttmann, L. (1976). *Spinal cord injuries. Comprehensive management and research* (2nd edn). Blackwell Scientific Publications, Oxford.

Guttmann, L. and Whitteridge, D. (1947). Effects of bladder distension on autonomic mechanisms after spinal cord injury. *Brain*, **70**, 371–404.

Guttmann, L., Frankel, H. L., and Paeslack, V. (1965). Cardiac irregularities during labour in paraplegic women. *Paraplegia*, **3**, 144–51.

Kooner, J. S., da Costa, D. F., Frankel, H. L., Bannister, R., Peart, W. S., and Mathias, C. J. (1987). Recumbency induces hypertension, diuresis and natriuresis in autonomic failure but diuresis alone in tetraplegia. *Journal of Hypertension*, **5** (suppl. 5), 327–9.

Lundberg, J. M., Saria, A., Franco-Cereceda, A., and Theodorsson-Norheim, E. (1985). Mechanisms underlying changes in the content of neuropeptide Y in cardiovascular nerves and adrenal gland induced by sympatholytic drugs. *Acta Physiologica Scandinavica*, **124**, 603–11.

Mathias, C. J. (1976a). Neurological disturbances of the cardiovascular system. D. Phil. thesis, University of Oxford.

Mathias, C. J. (1976b). Bradycardia and cardiac arrest during tracheal suction— mechanisms in tetraplegic patients. *European Journal of Intensive Care Medicine*, **2**, 137–56.

Mathias, C. J. (1987). Autonomic dysfunction. *British Journal of Hospital Medicine*, **38**, 238–43.

Mathias, C. J. and Frankel, H. L. (1983). Autonomic failure in tetraplegia. In Bannister, R., ed. *Autonomic failure: a textbook of clinical disorders of the autonomic nervous system* (ed. R. Bannister), pp. 453–88. Oxford University Press.

Mathias, C. J. and Frankel, H. L. (1983). Clinical manifestations of malfunctioning sympathetic mechanisms in tetraplegic man. *Journal of the Autonomic Nervous System*, **7**, 303–12.

Mathias, C. J. and Frankel, H. L. (1986). The neurological and hormonal control of blood vessels and heart in spinal man. *Journal of the Autonomic Nervous System*, (suppl.), 457–64.

Mathias, C. J. and Frankel, H. L. (1988). Cardiovascular control in spinal man. *Annual Review of Physiology*, **50**, 577–92.

Mathias, C. J., Christensen, N. J., Corbett, J. L., Frankel, H. L., Goodwin, T. J., and Peart, W. S. (1975). Plasma catecholamines, plasma renin activity and plasma aldosterone in tetraplegic man, horizontal and tilted. *Clinical Science and Molecular Medicine*, **49**, 291–9.

Mathias, C. J., Christensen, N. J., Corbett, J. L., Frankel, H. L., and Spalding, J. M. K. (1976a). Plasma catecholamines during paroxysmal neurogenic hypertension in quadriplegic man. *Circulation Research*, **39**, 204–8.

Mathias, C. J., Frankel, H. L., Christensen, N. J., and Spalding, N. M. K. (1976b). Enhanced pressor response to noradrenaline in patients with cervical spinal cord transection. *Brain*, **99**, 757–70.

Mathias, C. J., Christensen, N. J., Frankel, H. L., and Spalding, N. M. K. (1979a). Cardiovascular control in recently injured tetraplegics in spinal shock. *Quarterly Journal of Medicine*, NS, **48**, 273–9.

Mathias, C. J., Reid, J. L., Wing, L. M. H., Frakel, H. L., and Christensen, N. J. (1979b). Antihypertensive effects of clonidine in tetraplegic subjects devoid of central sympathetic control. *Clinical Science and Molecular Medicine*, **57**, 425–8s.

Mathias, C. J., Christensen, N. J., Frankel, H. L., and Peart, W. S. (1980). Renin release during head-up tilt occurs independently of sympathetic nervous activity in tetraplegic man. *Clinical Science*, **59**, 251–6.

Mathias, C. J., May, C. N., and Taylor, G. M. (1984). The renin–angiotensin system and hypertension—basic and clinical aspects. In *Molecular medicine*, Vol. 1 (ed. A. D. B. Malcolm), pp. 177–208. IRL Press, Oxford and Washington DC.

Mathias, C. J., Fosbraey, P., da Costa, D., Thornley, A. and Bannister, R. (1986). Desmopressin reduces nocturnal polyuria, reverses overnight weight loss and improves morning postural hypotension in autonomic failure. *British Medical Journal*, **293**, 353–4.

Meinecke, F. W., Rosenkranz, K. A., and Kurel, C. M. (1971). Regulation of the cardiovascular system in patients with fresh injuries to the spinal cord, preliminary report. *Paraplegia*, **9**, 109–13.

Pledger, H. G. (1962). Disorders of temperature regulation in acute traumatic paraplegia. *Journal of Bone and Joint Surgery*, **44**B, 110–13.

Schumacher, G. A. and Guthrie, T. C. (1951). Studies on headaches: mechanisms of headache and observations on other effects induced by distension of the bladder and rectum in subjects with spinal cord injuries. *Archives of Neurology and Psychiatry*, **65**, 568–80.

Walsh, J. J. (1960). Cardiovascular complications in paraplegia. Proceedings of Scientific Meeting, International Stoke Mandeville Games, Rome, pp. 37–45.

Welply, N., Mathias, C. J., and Frankel, H. L. (1975). Circulatory reflexes in tetraplegics during artificial ventilation and during general anaesthesia. *Paraplegia*, **13**, 172–82.

7

Bladder management
G. J. Fellows

Rehabilitation: physical, occupational, and social, is the aim of management after spinal cord injury or disease. The management of the lower urinary tract is crucial, since poor treatment may lead to unacceptable morbidity or even to renal failure and premature death.

Historically there have been four overlapping phases of bladder management, as expectations of improved length and quality of life for the paralysed have risen.

Phase 1—No treatment offered: The oldest known medical document, the *Edwin Smith Surgical Papyrus* from the seventeenth century BC describes tetraplegia as 'an ailment not to be treated' (Breasted 1930).

Phase 2—Permanent indwelling catheter: This was, and occasionally still is, appropriate when no attempt at rehabilitation is to be made—for example, in a patient with advanced malignant disease with a life expectancy of a few weeks, and also when other methods are inappropriate.

Phase 3—Achieve low-pressure voiding but sacrifice continence: Between the two World Wars it became apparent that upper tract dilatation occurred in patients with obstructed micturition, and this risk could be lessened by surgery to the bladder outflow tract. Incontinence in the male could be managed by an external urine-collecting device. Transurethral sphincterotomy was first advocated for patients with sacral lesions, and was later found to be effective in promoting micturition in those with high cord injury (Ross *et al.* 1958). It is safer to have a bladder that empties to completion at low pressure than a high-pressure bladder with excessive residual urine.

Phase 4—Achieve both efficient bladder emptying and continence: This is now a realistic goal for many patients. It should be considered for every new patient with a spinal injury, and only abandoned if shown not to be feasible.

The management of the individual patient can be considered in four stages: 1. *Early management* from the moment of injury until definitive management is instituted or the patient is discharged from hospital. 2. *Intermediate management* from discharge from hospital until definitive management if the latter is delayed for any reason. 3. *Definitive management*. 4. *Urological surveillance*, which should be lifelong for all patients. Different methods of management may need to be introduced at any stage if complications arise.

Early management

First 48 hours

Urinary retention is usual after spinal cord injury at any level. During spinal shock there is a loss of reflex detrusor contractions. Electromyography shows persistent activity of the external urethral striated sphincter but not of the anal sphincter (Koyanagi *et al.* 1984). The patient may have serious associated injuries, and during the resuscitation period an accurate hour-by-hour urine output record will be required.

Either an indwelling urethral catheter or a fine-bore suprapubic catheter should be inserted and connected to a closed continuous drainage system. Bladder expression has been advocated to avoid catheterization and its attendant risk of urinary infection (Golding 1968). This is sometimes possible, particularly in children, but is associated with a high incidence of early and severe upper tract dilatation (Smith *et al.* 1972).

It is important to avoid overdistension, at this stage and subsequently. Overdistension can delay the onset of reflex contractions and diminish subsequent bladder contractility (Hinman 1976).

During early rehabilitation

Occasionally a decision can be made immediately after injury that the appropriate management will be a permanent indwelling catheter. An example would be an elderly tetraplegic female patient who would not be expected to transfer unaided. Such a patient's independence and dignity is enhanced by an indwelling catheter.

In other patients a decision about definitive management will be made during their rehabilitation period, and in the mean time their bladders can be managed in one of four ways.

Expression has been mentioned already, and its dangers have been stressed. If excessive force is applied not only will high pressures be transmitted to the kidney if vesico-ureteric reflux occurs, but also the bladder neck and posterior urethra become distended and incompetent.

Intermittent catheterization is the most commonly used method, and the standard against which other methods must be judged (Guttmann and Frankel 1966). When first introduced it dramatically reduced the incidence of urethritis, urethral trauma, and epididymitis seen with indwelling catheters. With a regimen of intermittent catheterization and antibiotic instillation 90 per cent of patients can be discharged catheter-free and with sterile urine (Pearman 1971; Ott and Rossier 1971). Catheterization can be performed by medical or nursing staff or trained orderlies until such time as patients can be trained to do it themselves. Particular care must be taken to use a sterile as opposed to a clean technique while in hospital, because there may be antibiotic-resistant organisms in the environment. A disadvantage of intermittent catheterization is that in order to avoid overdistension fluid intake is restricted. During the period of immobilization after injury hypercalciuria and hyperphosphaturia coupled with oliguria can lead to stone-formation (Burr 1978).

Fine-bore suprapubic catheters provide a feasible alternative method of management (Cook and Smith 1976; Namiki *et al.* 1978). A study in which patients were allocated at random to either fine-bore suprapubic or intermittent catheterization showed no difference between the two methods in regard to febrile episodes, incidence of urinary infections, time to establishment of reflex micturition, or final outcome (Grundy *et al.* 1983). Some patients found suprapubic catheters more acceptable, and they were cheaper and less time-consuming. They are, however, prone to fall out, and may block with debris. A high fluid intake should be maintained.

Indwelling urethral catheters have improved over the last twenty years since intermittent catheterization was introduced. Silicone- and teflon-coated catheters are relatively inert, and provoke little in the way of urethritis. In a retrospective non-randomized study the outcome one year after injury was the same whatever method of early bladder management was followed (Lloyd *et al.* 1986).

Decide definitive management

During the first few weeks after injury a decision should be made regarding definitive bladder-management. Bladder-voiding to completion with continence between voids is the ideal which should be considered in every case. Often the ideal is not practical or is unattainable. There are several less desirable forms of definitive management which may be adopted at this stage. Intermittent clean self-catheterization may be appropriate for the patient in retention. The male who can void but is incontinent may wear an external urine-collecting device of the condom urinal variety, whereas patients of both sexes may cope with a moderate degree of incontinence with pads. An indwelling urethral catheter or permanent suprapubic catheter may occasionally be appropriate, particularly for those with a short prognosis.

The following factors are taken into consideration when deciding definitive management:

(a) Prognosis. Is life expectancy a matter of weeks, months, years, or decades?

(b) Sex of the patient. In the female, it is imperative to maintain continence because of the unsatisfactory nature of external urine-collecting devices.

(c) General factors. Will the patient be able to transfer from wheelchair to toilet? Will there be adequate assistance in the home? Has he or she the manual dexterity and clarity of vision to perform self-catheterization or to operate the control mechanism of an artificial sphincter? Does spasm preclude these manœuvres? Is urine leakage threatening the skin?

(d) Pre-existing disease of the urinary tract. In most young patients the urinary tract will be normal. The older male may have prostatic hyperplasia, and occasionally other conditions such as urological malignancies will be encountered.

(e) Sexual function in the male. Does the patient have erections? Can he ejaculate? Does he hope to have a family? How important is it to preserve sexual function in this particular individual?

(f) Neuro-urological status. The behaviour of the lower urinary tract must be determined by urodynamic studies. These have been discussed in an earlier chapter and will not be described in detail now. They include filling cystometry, pressure/flow studies, urethral pressure profilometry, electromyography, and imaging of the lower urinary tract by radiology or ultrasound (Fig. 7.1) (Thomas *et al.* 1975; Perkash and Friedland 1986; Fellows *et al.* 1987).

(g) Autonomic dysreflexia. Occasionally severe dysreflexia secondary to high bladder pressures and detrusor sphincter dyssynergia will necessitate surgery to the bladder outflow tract (Barton *et al.* 1986).

(h) Patient preference. Often issues are not clear-cut, and there may be more than one feasible method of management. For the rest of his life the patient must take his full share of responsibility for his welfare, and he must understand the methods of bladder management which are available to him. He may express a strong preference, which should be respected.

(i) Potential for neurological recovery. If recovery of function is likely then destructive or irreversible procedures should be avoided. Recovery is most likely when the lesion is incomplete, and may continue for eighteen months to two years after injury. After the return of lower limb reflexes in patients with suprasacral cord injury the bladder may occasionally be areflexic on filling cystometry. This may be due to a second cord lesion involving the sacral segments; but if the bulbo-cavernosus reflex and pelvic floor EMG are normal then bladder reflex activity is likely to return, and definitive treatment should be delayed (Light *et al.* 1985).

Intermediate management

If for any reason definitive management is delayed some form of medium-term management must be instituted. The most usual reason for this delay is waiting for possible neurological recovery. Other reasons include severe associated injury requiring prolonged treatment, pregnancy or impending puberty, and transfer to another hospital for definitive management.

Intermittent clean self-catheterization is a suitable regimen (Lapides *et al.* 1972). It is associated with fewer infective complications, calculi, or cases of

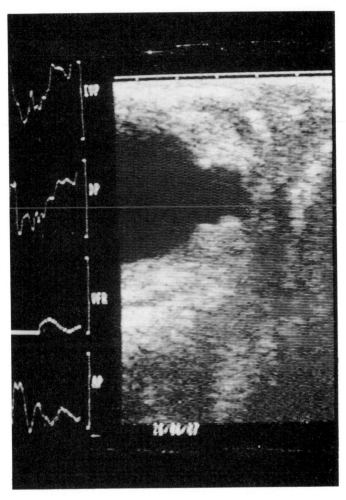

Fig. 7.1. Videocystometry with ultrasound imaging of bladder and posterior urethra.

urethral trauma than indwelling catheters. It is suitable for both male and female patients (McGuire and Savastano 1983). It can be continued as definitive treatment.

Indwelling urethral or suprapubic catheters may also enable the patient and clinician to 'buy time', but should only be used if intermittent self-catheterization is not feasible. Techniques and complications of intermittent and indwelling catheters are described later.

Definitive management

There are five different methods of management:

1. *Voiding with continence between voids*

Voiding may be by volitional activation of the voiding reflex, by triggering the reflex by abdominal tapping or some other manœuvre (Glahn 1970), by abdominal straining, or by an implanted electrical nerve stimulator such as the Brindley anterior sacral root stimulator (Brindley *et al.* 1982). Continence depends on a competent sphincter mechanism. An incompetent sphincter may be replaced with an artificial sphincter.

2. *Intermittent self-catheterization with continence*

This method is suitable for both sexes if the patient is unable to pass urine or has a large residual volume and is able to remain continent for a minimum of 3 hours. Infection or upper tract dilatation are not contraindications.

3. *Voiding with incontinence between voids*

Voiding may occur by any of the means listed under 1. A patient with a minor degree of incontinence may manage with pads. A male who can wear a condom urine-collecting device can tolerate a much greater degree of incontinence.

If the penis is too small to hold a condom urinal it can be lengthened and stiffened with a simple type of non-inflatable penile implant, and then a condom can be applied easily.

4. *Indwelling urethral or suprapubic catheter*

The complications of indwelling catheters are numerous, and include ascending urinary infection, prostatitis, epididymitis, urethritis, periurethral abscess, urethral fistulae and diverticula, calculi, contracted bladder, catheters blocked with debris, bypassing, urethral erosion, and catheter extrusion. Despite these hazards an indwelling catheter is preferable to intractable incontinence in the female or the occasional male who cannot wear a condom urinal.

5. *Urinary diversion*

This is reserved for the female patient with severe incontinence who cannot retain a catheter on account of severe urethral erosion and a contracted hyperreflexic bladder in whom lesser procedures have failed. Such patients are grateful to be rendered dry. Options include a suprapubic catheter with formal closure of the urethra (Feneley 1983) and ilial conduit (Malone *et al.* 1985).

Choice of definitive management

Methods 4 or 5 are usually reserved for when other methods have failed. A decision must be made whether to discourage voiding, concentrate on maintaining continence, and rely on self-catheterization or to strive for complete bladder-emptying at low pressure and then aim to achieve continence. The greater the degree of detrusor hyperreflexia the greater the likelihood of incontinence between voids making intermittent self-catheterization unsatisfactory.

In the female greater effort will be expended in minimizing detrusor hyperreflexia in order to preserve continence, whereas in the male more attention will be paid to lowering outflow resistance and thus lowering intravesical pressure. The incidence of upper tract dilatation secondary to detrusor sphincter dyssynergia is much greater in males than females.

Male patients with cauda equinal lesions who can walk often have difficulty keeping a condom urinal in position. They benefit from the insertion of an artificial sphincter.

Patients of both sexes with suprasacral lesions, particularly with incomplete bladder-emptying and recurrent urinary infections, are suitable for anterior sacral root stimulation. If detrusor hyperreflexia is severe the posterior sacral roots may be divided. The role of artificial sphincters and anterior sacral root stimulators will be considered in more detail later.

Procedures to promote voiding

Patients' manœuvres

When the detrusor is areflexic, or when bladder contractions fade away before the bladder is empty voiding may be encouraged by raising the intra-abdominal pressure by straining or leaning with both fists on the lower abdomen or on a small firm cushion pressing into it.

Detrusor contractions may be triggered by stimulating the penis or inner thigh, but most successfully by a series of sharp taps on the suprapubic region.

Many patients find they empty their bladders more efficiently when they have a bowel action. If the patient inserts one or two gloved fingers into the anal canal and pulls backwards steadily until he feels the anal sphincter relax the external urethral sphincter relaxes simultaneously, and he can void by abdominal straining (Low and Donovan 1981).

Drugs

Drugs to increase detrusor contractions

Parasympathomimetic agents such as carbachol, bethanechol, and distigmine bromide have been widely used. Bethanechol can be given orally (50 mg qds) or subcutaneously (5–10 mg). Although capable of causing contraction of detrusor muscle strips *in vitro* there is very little evidence that it can improve bladder emptying *in vivo* (Light and Scott 1983; Blaivas 1984).

Intravesical instillations of prostaglandin E_2 are reported to enhance bladder contractions in those with intact sacral reflex arcs (Desmond *et al.* 1980). In a double-blind placebo-controlled study of prostaglandin F_2 alpha for patients in retention three days ater surgery for stress incontinence, 15/18 in the prostaglandin group voided, whereas 0/18 in the placebo group managed to pass urine (Tammela *et al.* 1987). Others have noted no response to prostaglandin instillations (Delaere *et al.* 1981).

The role of sympathetic innervation on detrusor action is disputed. In the intact individual sympathetic activity inhibits bladder-contraction; but this action may be reversed in patients with suprasacral injury, when alpha blocking agents appear sometimes to promote bladder-contraction (Mathe *et al.* 1985). Others have noted detrusor inhibition with phentolamine (Thomas *et al.* 1984). A neurohistological study of bladder-wall biopsies from patients with cord injury failed to show any increase in noradrenergic nerves in high lesion patients (Nordling *et al.* 1980).

Drugs to lower bladder outflow resistance

Smooth muscle at the bladder neck and posterior urethra, more developed in the male than female, has a rich adrenergic nerve supply (Gosling and Dixon 1975). Patients with cauda equina lesions may show obstruction at the level of the membranous urethra due to contraction of smooth muscle at this level (Abel *et al.* 1974; Koyanagi *et al.* 1982). Alpha adrenergic blockade can reduce outflow resistance and promote bladder-emptying (Krane and Olsson 1973). Varying clinical success with alpha adrenolytic agents has been reported (Mobley 1976; Hachen 1980). Thomas *et al.* failed to demonstrate any decrease in outflow resistance by phentolamine (Thomas *et al.* 1984).

Phenoxybenzamine has been the most widely used alpha adrenolytic drug. Reports of gastrointestinal tumours in rats given phenoxybenzamine have directed attention to other alpha adrenolytic agents. Prazosin, an alpha-1 antagonist, is an effective alternative drug. Initial dose should be low, and care should be taken to avoid postural hypotension. Indoramin has similar action.

Spasticity of the pelvic floor will prevent the normal descent of the bladder at the start of micturition. In addition bladder-emptying may be impaired by detrusor/striated sphincter dyssynergia. Although some improvement in bladder-emptying with striated muscle relaxants such as baclofen at high dosage has been reported (Florante *et al.* 1980), their use in treating dys-synergia in other hands has been disappointing (Hachen and Kruckner 1977).

Bladder outflow surgery

The objective is to lower outflow resistance, and surgery should be limited to the portion of the outflow tract where the obstruction lies. In the majority of male patients with either sacral or suprasacral cord lesions this is in the infra-montanal membranous portion of the urethra. Bladder-outflow surgery in the female is rarely required or performed because of the risk of incontin-ence. Occasionally flow is obstructed at the bladder neck, and it should not be forgotten that the older man may suffer from benign prostatic hyperplasia or prostatic carcinoma. The level of obstruction can be seen clearly by video cysto-urethrography or transrectal ultrasonography (Nordling *et al.* 1982; Perkash and Friedland 1986). Most operations are endoscopic, and open operations are very rarely required.

Internal membranous urethrotomy (sphincterotomy)

The value of this operation in facilitating bladder-emptying is well estab-lished (Gibbon 1974). An incision is made from the verumontanum to the bulbous urethra with a Collings knife electrode or resectoscope loop through all muscular tissue until the plane of venous sinuses is reached. Because of the proximity of the nervi erigentes the incidence of post-operative erectile impotence is less (but still significant) if the incision is made in the antero-median (12 o'clock) direction rather than laterally (Philp *et al.* 1983). Following complete division of the distal sphincter mechanism (smooth and striated) the characteristic peak of high pressure on a static urethral pressure profile is absent (Abel *et al.* 1975).

Bladder-neck incision or resection

It is clearly inappropriate to incise the bladder neck if this region is noted to open widely on imaging studies. Bladder-neck surgery may be necessary when failure to void follows a sphincterotomy. It may be combined with sphincterotomy, particularly in patients with high lesions and vesico-ureteric reflux, when it is imperative to lower outflow resistance to a minimum and incontinence and retrograde ejaculation are unimportant (Ruutu and Lehtonen 1985). Repeat operations after sphincterotomy or bladder-neck resection are required in about a third of cases (O'Flynn 1976; Fellows *et al.* 1977).

Nerve stimulation

Intraluminal electrical stimulation of the bladder was reported to induce detrusor contractions in neuropathic bladders (Katona and Eckstein 1974). Subsequent experience failed to confirm these results (Nicholas and Eckstein 1975). Direct electrical stimulation of the detrusor with implanted electrodes has only met with very limited success. Better results were obtained with direct stimulus of the conus via implanted electrodes (Grimes and Nashold 1974).

Anterior sacral root stimulation

Inadequate, unsustained detrusor contractions are a more important reason for incomplete emptying in patients with suprasacral lesions than is detrusor sphincter dyssynergia. Anterior sacral root stimulation is a logical concept to provide efferent stimulation of sufficient strength and duration to ensure complete emptying of the bladder (Brindley 1977).

The anterior roots of S_2 and S_3 and, if indicated by peroperative cystometry, S_4 are placed within electrodes connected to a subcutaneous receiver placed in the chest wall, which is activated by a hand-held transmitter capable of variable stimulus strength, duration, and wave-form (Fig. 7.2). Severe hyperreflexia can be abolished by concomitant section of S_2 and S_3 posterior roots. The device stimulates the detrusor, the external sphincter, and the pelvic floor. The stimulus is applied in bursts, and micturition usually occurs between bursts, when the striated muscles relax but the detrusor continues to contract. The clinical result is usually a diminution of residual urine, increase in functional capacity, improvement in continence, and fewer urinary infections (Cardozo *et al.* 1984). The insertion of an anterior sacral root stimulator involves a major operation. Work is in progress to develop a method of stimulating sacral nerves by means of a wire inserted percutaneously into the epidural space, thus avoiding major surgery. If shown to be effective this could be inserted very soon after injury.

Procedures to promote continence

Incontinence may be due to detrusor hyperreflexia, sphincter incompetence, or both.

Drugs

Drugs to inhibit bladder contractions

Most of the motor innervation of the bladder in man is cholinergic (Kinder and Mundy 1985), and the main drugs to inhibit detrusor contractions are, therefore, anti-cholinergic drugs. Unfortunately, side-effects from general

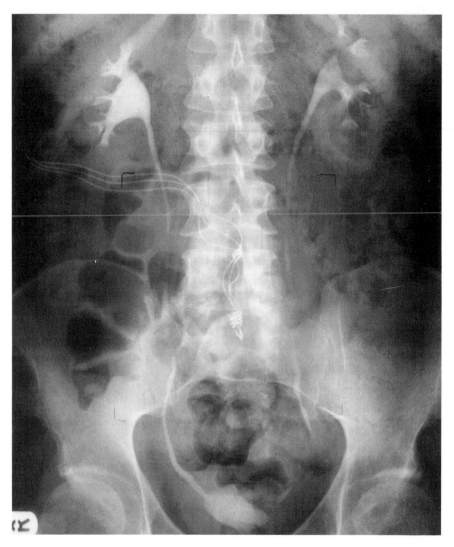

Fig. 7.2. Intravenous urogram showing position of electrodes of a Brindley anterior
sacral root stimulator

anti-muscarinic actions (dry mouth, blurred vision, tachycardia, and constipation) limit the dosage which can be tolerated. Propantheline is the most
widely prescribed drug. It should be administered in as high a dose as can be
tolerated. Emepomium bromide and flavoxate hydrochloride are also given.
More recently oxybutynin has been available and is a highly potent agent
(Moisey *et al.* 1980).

Tricyclic antidepressants (for example, imipramine) decrease bladder contractility and also increase outlet resistance by an alpha adrenergic action (Cole and Fried 1972).

Calcium antagonists such as nifedipine and terodiline diminish detrusor contractility and also increase outlet resistance by an alpha-adrenergic action unproven (Gerstenberg *et al.* 1986). If prostaglandins stimulate bladder contractions, then prostaglandin inhibitors might influence bladder behaviour. If they have any action it appears to be weak (Cardozo *et al.* 1980).

Drugs to increase outlet resistance

The mild alpha-adrenergic action of impramine has been mentioned. Other alpha stimulants include ephedrine and phenylpropanolamine. Ephedrine raises the maximum urethral closure pressure, and reduces incontinence in some patients. Phenylpropanolamine is a component of several proprietary preparations for allergic rhinitis and the common cold. It has a clinical application in sphincteric weakness (Montague and Stewart 1979). Alpha stimulant drugs can cause a rise in blood-pressure, insomnia, anxiety, palpitations, and other symptoms of central nervous system stimulation.

In practice it is appropriate to give drugs in combination—for example, oxybutynin to decrease detrusor contractions and phenylpropanolamine to increase outflow resistance. Controlled clinical trials of different drug combinations are lacking. Wein has reviewed the action of drugs on the lower urinary tract (Wein 1987).

Nerve stimulation and division

Detrusor activity can be inhibited reflexly by stimulating appropriate afferent nerves, including the posterior tibial, peroneal, pudendal, and sacral roots (McGuire *et al.* 1983; Vodusek *et al.* 1986). The clinical application of these techniques is awaited.

An attempt can be made to denervate the bladder by interrupting its motor nerve supply at various sites (Torrens 1985). These include division of sacral anterior nerve roots (Hald and Hebjorn 1978) (or posterior roots to break the reflex arc), selective nerve blocks at the sacral foramina (Allousi *et al.* 1984), division of nerves via transvaginal, transabdominal, or parasacral approaches, subtrigonal phenol blockade (Ewing *et al.* 1982), and bladder transsection. The more proximal the nerve division the more is denervated in addition to the bladder—for example, the anal sphincter. A problem with all denervation procedures is nerve regeneration and a return of detrusor hyper-reflexia, possibly due to the formation of local reflex arcs. Very variable results of nerve ablation procedures have been reported.

Bladder transsection may be by open operation (Hindmarsh *et al.* 1977) or endoscopic (Parsons *et al.* 1984). The open operation is more certain in its result than endoscopic transsection (Lucas and Thomas 1987).

Subtrigonal phenol blockade of the pelvic plexuses is often effective, and can be repeated (Blackford *et al.* 1984).

Prolonged bladder distension

Ideopathic detrusor instability can be abolished by prolonged bladder distension (Dunn *et al.* 1974). The mechanism is unknown. Good results in the initial series have not been repeated (Pengelly *et al.* 1978). In an attempt to prevent detrusor hyperreflexia and to enable patients with cord injuries to remain dry on a regimen of intermittent self-catheterization Iwatsubo *et al.* encouraged overdistension of the bladder soon after injury to a volume of about 1000 ml (Iwatsubo *et al.* 1984).

Augmentation cystoplasty

Small-volume high-pressure bladders can be converted to high-volume low-pressure bladders by augmentation cystoplasty. If the bladder volume is greatly reduced and the bladder wall very thickened the fundus should be excised, and the bladder should be reconstructed with caecum or colon. If the bladder can be filled to about 150 ml it is possible to perform a 'clam' cystoplasty (Mundy and Stephenson 1985). The bladder is bivalved in a coronal or sagittal plane, and a length of ileum, opened along its anti-mesenteric border, interposed between the two halves of the bladder. After an augmentation cystoplasty the bladder is emptied by abdominal straining or intermittent self-catheterization.

Surgery to increase outflow resistance

Periuretheral Teflon injection (Schulman et al. 1984)

The injection of Teflon endoscopically to build up the tissue around the bladder neck may prevent incontinence due to sphincter weakness.

Endoscopic bladder-neck suspension (Stamey 1973)

Bladder-neck suspension can prevent incontinence in female patients provided intravesical pressures are not too high (Kato *et al.* 1987).

Urethral reconstruction

Female patients with severe urethral erosion from indwelling catheters and incontinence or leakage around their catheters present a problem. Reconstruction of the vaginal urethra merely lengthens the urethra without improving continence (Gunst *et al.* 1987). Bladder-neck suspension may succeed, and a simultaneous urethral reconstruction to advance the meatus will make subsequent self-catheterization easier. When the bladder is of adequate capacity an intra-abdominal urethra may be constructed out of full-thickness bladder wall by a variety of techniques (Gunst *et al.* 1987).

Artificial urinary sphincter

Different designs of artificial sphincter have been developed, the most widely accepted being the Brantley Scott device (Scott *et al.* 1974). It has been used extensively to treat neurogenic urinary incontinence due to sphincter incompetence. In the male a preliminary sphincterotomy is necessary. The device is entirely implanted, and consists of an inflatable cuff placed around the bladder neck or the membranous or bulbous urethra, a reservoir alongside the bladder, and a pump control-mechanism in the scrotum or labium majus. The components are connected with silicone tubing (Fig. 7.3).

The patient transfers fluid from the cuff to the reservoir by squeezing the control pump, and can then pass urine by abdominal straining. The cuff automatically fills again to a predetermined pressure. Low bladder-pressures are a prerequisite for the successful use of an artificial sphincter. A small proportion of patients with atonic bladders convert to having hyperreflexic bladders after insertion of a sphincter (Jakobsen and Hald 1986). Denervation supersensitivity provides a possible explanation. Over a third of patients require revisionary surgery, and in some there is a minor degree of permanent incontinence. Nevertheless, in the majority the results are excellent and the patients satisfied (Heathcote *et al.* 1987).

Surveillance programme

In the long-term care of the paraplegic, careful and regular clinical assessment of the urinary tract is essential (England and Low 1985). The main reason for lifelong surveillance is that complications can arise even after years of apparently stable function. The patient's neurological status may change—for example, with the development of a syrinx. The older man may develop prostatic hyperplasia. The prepubertal boy as he enters puberty may develop obstruction due to detrusor sphincter dyssynergia as the external striated sphincter hypertrophies. The upper urinary tracts may dilate even in the absence of vesico-ureteric reflux.

The patient is always at risk of developing urinary infections, with all the complications which might follow. Calculi, both renal and vesical, are a result of hypercalcuria and infection. Catheters and appliances bring numerous complications in their train. Absence of normal sensation means that many conditions can develop unnoticed by the patient, which makes their diagnosis more difficult in the paraplegic, and is a cogent reason for regular assessment by the clinician even in the absence of symptoms.

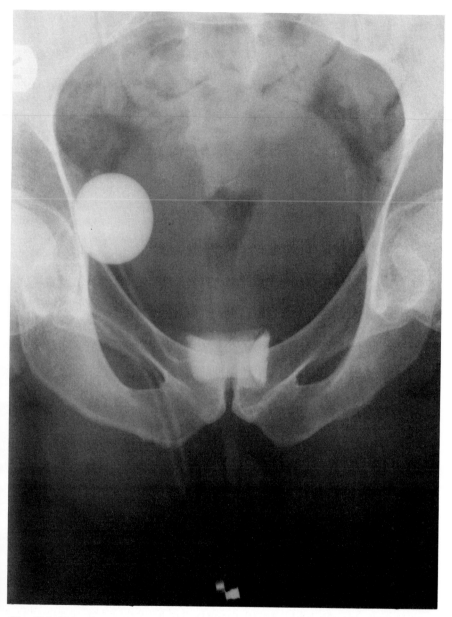

Fig. 7.3. Brantley–Scott AS 800 artificial sphincter *in situ* showing cuff around bladder-neck, balloon reservoir to right of bladder, and control pump in right side of scrotum.

Frequency of follow-up

No hard and fast rules can be applied as to the frequency of follow-up visits. There may be reasons for frequent out-patient attendance unrelated to the urinary tract. Complications in the urinary tract may necessitate frequent attendance. In the absence of any particular complications the well, rehabilitated patient should be seen annually. The patient's own General Practitioner should play an active role, but should not replace the annual visit to a spinal injuries unit.

The routine check-up

When there are no known urological complications this should consist of a history, physical examination (which should include blood-pressure measurement, rectal examination, and neurological assessment), urine microscopy and culture, haemoglobin, urea, and electrolyte estimation. If ultrasound facilities are available in the out-patient clinic an approximate assessment can be made of residual urine volume (Kiely *et al.* 1987) and of the degree of dilatation of the upper urinary tracts. More detailed information on the upper tracts can be obtained with either intravenous urography (IVU) or renal isotope scans. The main upper-tract complications are calculi and hydronephrosis. These can be virtually excluded by a plain abdominal X-ray and an ultrasound scan. An IVU is necessary to show fine detail of upper-tract anatomy. An isotope scan reveals renal function rather than anatomy, although it will demonstrate moderate degrees of dilatation. It is suggested that ultrasound scans are conducted every one to three years in males and less frequently in females, as the risk of upper-tract deterioration is lower in female subjects.

Urodynamic studies, because of their invasive nature and cost, should be reserved for specific indications. These include the development of new lower urinary tract symptoms, such as increasing difficulty voiding or incontinence, and upper-tract dilatation or increasing residual urine volume.

Flexible cystoscopy is now an established out-patient procedure. Cystoscopy, flexible or rigid, should be done to answer specific questions, and not as routine.

The patient's responsibility

Every adult who is free of major psychiatric illness should be responsible for maintaining his own bodily health to the best of his ability. This responsibility is not diminished if he has a chronic disability, but rather is increased. The fostering of such a responsible attitude is an important aspect of his rehabilitation, and enables him to gain independence and increased self-respect (England and Low 1985).

Bodily functions which previously required little conscious thought and no effort may be so altered that their satisfactory execution requires retraining of the patient in new techniques. For instance he may be unaware of a full bladder, and will need to time his acts of micturition by the clock. He must be taught to empty his bladder as completely as possible on every occasion, and he should know the reason for this. He will require training in self-catheterization, the use of his artificial sphincter or sacral root stimulator, or the correct way to manage a condom urinal or indwelling catheter. By attention to detail many urological complications can be avoided. Also by close self-observation the patient may notice the first signs of complications arising and report them immediately. This constant self-observation, which in an uninjured patient would amount to hypochondria, is essential to maintain his health.

Urological complications

The kidney and ureter do not require an innervation—hence the feasibility of renal transplantation. The bladder and urethra are dependent upon the central nervous system, and almost all urological complications in paraplegia are a direct consequence of disordered function of the lower urinary tract. This chapter has, therefore, concentrated on this disordered function; but the account would be incomplete without brief notes on the more common complications which might ensue. The reader is directed to standard urological texts for more detail.

Upper-tract dilatation

Hydronephrosis/hydroureter can occur silently soon or many years after injury. It is usually due to bladder outflow tract obstruction, even when unilateral or associated with vesico-ureteric reflux. Relief of obstruction often leads to its resolution. Upper-tract dilatation may be due to impacted ureteric calculi, or occasionally to ureteric obstruction within the wall of a hypertrophied bladder.

The need to correct reflux is a matter of debate. It is important to convert high-pressure to low-pressure reflux by attention to the detrusor and/or the urethral sphincters. The combination of intermittent self-catheterization and reflux may carry an increased risk for the kidney. Reimplantation of the ureter into a trabeculated bladder is difficult, and reflux in such instances can be prevented by endoscopic juxta-urethral injection of teflon paste.

Urinary infection

It is almost universal for urinary infection to develop at some time. The usual organisms are bowel flora, and the method of entry by urethral catheters. Most patients rendered free of catheters will have sterile urine.

In some patients infections prove difficult to eradicate despite the correction as far as possible of voiding dysfunction, attention to personal hygiene, a high fluid intake, and frequent voiding. It is better to accept a low-grade persistent asymptomatic infection than to give repeated courses of different antibiotics and produce resistant organisms.

Infection may spread to the genital tract—commonly the prostate and epididymis—particularly when an indwelling catheter is worn. Acute febrile episodes within the first few months of injury may be attacks of bacteraemia or, more often, endotoxaemia without viable organisms in the bloodstream.

Calculi

High excretion rates of calcium and phosphate after injury predispose to calculus formation—hence the importance of a high fluid intake. Calculi in the upper urinary tract are usually infective in origin, and secondary to *Proteus* urinary infections. Bladder calculi form on the balloons of Foley catheters, and may then grow in a sump of residual urine. Renal stones can be treated by extracorporeal shock-wave lithotripsy of percutaneous nephrolithotomy, as well as by open operation.

Renal failure

The incidence of renal failure as a cause of death is falling, but is still higher than in the general population. A combination of urinary obstruction or reflux with infection and often with calculi leads to chronic pyelonephritis. Acute pyonephrosis due to obstructive ureteric calculi can rapidly destroy a kidney, and pain may be absent if the cord lesion is above the mid-thoracic level. Another course of renal failure is amyloidosis secondary to chronically infected urine or pressure sores.

Autonomic dysreflexia (see Chapter 6)

Afferent stimuli from the bladder, particularly when intravesical pressure is high, as in detrusor/sphincter dyssynergia, can trigger an attack of autonomic dysreflexia. This is characterized by sweating at about the level of the cord lesion, flushing above the lesion, sudden hypertension (giving rise to severe headache), and bradycardia. These phenomena are secondary to excessive uninhibited sympathetic discharge below the cord lesion (Mathias and Frankel 1983). The condition may be alleviated by preventing high intravesical pressure—for instance, by sphincterotomy to lower bladder outflow resistance.

Urethral damage from catheters

In the absence of sensation severe pressure necrosis of the urethra can be inflicted by catheters. If the catheter is taped to the thigh, pressure is applied to the floor of the urethra at the peno-scrotal junction. This may lead to periurethral abscesses, diverticula, and fistulae. The risk is minimized by taping the catheter to the abdominal wall.

In both sexes severe urethral erosion may occur. In the female the whole urethra is sometimes destroyed, and bladder epithelium is clearly visible on external inspection. In the male the external meatus extends ventrally along the shaft of the penis. The balloon of the Foley catheter may be inflated within the urethra, causing urethral rupture and extravasation of urine.

Carcinoma of the bladder

Bladder cancer, usually squamous carcinoma, may arise ten or more years after cord injury. The risk is at least twenty times that in the general population (El Masri and Fellows 1981).

Conclusion

Better urological care over the last few decades has led to a lower risk of death from renal failure, a lower incidence of calculi, and less urethral damage from indwelling catheters. The physiology of micturition is better understood, although there is still much to learn; and this has led to more effective pharmacological regulation of the lower urinary tract.

The rediscovery of intermittent self-catheterization and surgical advances with artificial sphincters and anterior sacral root stimulators have enabled many patients to be continent. The dream of normal, or something approaching normal, micturition can frequently now be a reality. The prime aim remains the preservation of renal function, and the achievement of continence must never put the kidneys at risk.

References

Abel, B. J., Gibbon, N. O. K., Jameson, R. M., and Krishnan, K. R. (1974). The neuropathic urethra. *Lancet*, **2**, 1229–30.

Abel, B. J., Ross, C. J., Gibbon, N. O. K., and Jameson, R. M. (1975). Urethral pressure measurement after division of the external sphincter. *Paraplegia*, **13**, 37–41.

Allousi, S., Loew, F., Mast, G. J., Alzin, H., and Wolf, D. (1984). Treatment of detrusor instability of the urinary bladder by selective sacral blockage. *British Journal of Urology*, **56**, 464–7.

Barton, C. H., Khonsari, F., Vaziri, N. D., Byrne, C., Gordon, S., and Friis, R. (1986). The effect of modified transurethral sphincterotomy on autonomic dysreflexia. *Journal of Urology*, **135**, 83–5.

Breasted, J. H. (1930). *The Edwin Smith surgical papyrus*, Vol. 1, pp. 316–42. University of Chicago Press.

Blackford, H. N., Murray, K., Stephenson, T. P., and Mundy, A. R. (1984). Results of transvesical infiltration of the pelvic plexuses with phenol in 116 patients. *British Journal of Urology*, **56**, 647–9.

Blaivas, J. (1984). If you currently prescribe bethanechol chloride for urinary retention, please raise your hand. *Neurourology and Urodynamics*, **3**, 209–10.

Brindley, G. S. (1977). An implant to empty the bladder or close the urethra. *Journal of Neurology, Neurosurgery and Psychiatry*, **40**, 358–69.

Brindley, G. S., Polkey, C. E., and Rushton, D. N. (1982). Sacral anterior root stimulators for bladder control in paraplegia. *Paraplegia*, **20**, 365–81.

Burr, R. G. (1978). A relationship between the composition of the urine and that of urinary tract calculi in spinal patients. *Paraplegia*, **16**, 59–64.

Cardozo, L., Stanton, S., and Robinson, H. (1980). Evaluation of flurbiprofen in detrusor instability. *British Medical Journal*, **280**, 281–2.

Cardozo, L., Krishnan, K. R., Polkey, C. E., Rushton, D. N., and Brindley G. S. (1984). Urodynamic observations on patients with sacral anterior root stimulators. *Paraplegia*, **22**, 201–9.

Cole, A. and Fried, F. (1972). Favourable experiences with imipramine in the treatment of neuropathic bladder. *Journal of Urology*, **107**, 44–5.

Cook, J. B. and Smith, P. H. (1976). Percutaneous suprapubic cystostomy after spinal cord injury. *British Journal of Urology*, **48**, 119–21.

Delaere, K. P. J., Thomas, C. M. G., Moonen, W. A., and Debruyne, F. M. J. (1981). The value of intravesical Prostaglandin E_2 and F_2 alpha in women with abnormalities of bladder emptying. *British Journal of Urology*, **53**, 306–9.

Desmond, A. D., Bultitude, M. I., Hills, N. H., and Shuttleworth, K. E. D. (1980). Clinical experience with intravesical prostaglandin E_2. *British Journal of Urology*, **52**, 357–66.

Dunn, M., Smith, J. C., and Ardran, G. M. (1974). Prolonged bladder distension as a treatment of urgency and urge incontinence of urine. *British Journal of Urology*, **46**, 645–52.

El-Masri, W. S. and Fellows, G. J. (1981). Bladder cancer after spinal cord injury. *Paraplegia*, **19**, 265–70.

England, E. J. and Low, A. I. (1985). Long-term management and prevention of urinary tract disease. In *Lifetime care of the paraplegic patient* (ed. G. M. Bedbrook), pp. 94–108. Churchill Livingstone, Edinburgh.

Ewing, R., Bultitude, M. I., and Shuttleworth K. E. D. (1982). Subtrigonal phenol injection for urge incontinence secondary to detrusor instability in females. *British Journal of Urology*, **54**, 689–92.

Fellows, G. J., Nuseibeh, I., and Walsh, J. J. (1977). Choice of operation to promote micturition after spinal cord injury. *British Journal of Urology*, **59**, 218–21.

Fellows, G. J., Cannell, L. B., and Ravichandran, G. (1987). Transrectal ultrasonography compared with voiding cystourethrography after spinal cord injury. *British Journal of Urology*, **49**, 721–4.

Feneley, R. C. L. (1983). The management of female incontinence by suprapubic catheterization with or without urethral closure. *British Journal of Urology*, **55**, 203–7.

Florante, J., Leyson, J., Martin, B. F., and Sporer, A. (1980). Baclofen in the treatment of detrusor–sphincter dyssynergia in spinal cord injury patients. *Journal of Urology*, **124**, 82–4.

Gerstenberg, T. C., Klarskov, P., Ramirez, D., and Hald, T. (1986). Terodiline in the treatment of women with urgency and motor urge incontinence. *British Journal of Urology*, **58**, 129–33.

Gibbon, N. O. K. (1974). Neurogenic bladder in spinal cord injury. Management of patients in Liverpool, England. *Urological Clinics of North America*, **1**(1), 147–54.

Glahn, B. E. (1970). Manual provocation of micturition contraction in neurogenic bladders. *Scandinavian Journal of Urology and Nephrology*, **4**, 25–36.

Golding, J. S. R. (1968). Early management of traumatic paraplegia in males. *Rehabilitation*, **66**, 49–53.

Gosling, J. A. and Dixon, J. S. (1975). The structure and innervation of smooth muscle in the wall of the bladder neck and proximal urethra. *British Journal of Urology*, **47**, 549–58.

Grimes, J. H. and Nashold, B. S. (1974). Clinical application of electronic bladder stimulation in paraplegics. *British Journal of Urology*, **46**, 653–7.

Grundy, D. J., Fellows, G. J., Nuseibeh, I., Gillett, A. P., and Silver, J. R. (1983). A comparison of fine-bore suprapubic and an intermittent urethral catheterisation regime after spinal cord injury. *Paraplegia*, **21**, 227–32.

Gunst, M. A., Ackerman, D., and Zingg, E. J. (1987). Urethral reconstruction in females. *European Urology*, **13**, 62–9.

Guttmann, L. and Frankel, H. (1966). The value of intermittent catheterisation in the early management of traumatic paraplegia and tetraplegia. *Paraplegia*, **4**, 63–83.

Hachen, H. J. (1980). Clinical and urodnaic assessment of alpha adrenolytic therapy in patients with neurogeic bladder dysfunction. *Paraplegia*, **18**, 229–38.

Hachen, H. J. and Kruckner, V. (1977). Clinical and laboratory assessment of the efficacy of baclofen (lioresal) on urethral sphincter spasticity in patients with traumatic paraplegia. *European Urology*, **3**, 237–40.

Hald, T. and Hebjorn, S. (1978). Results of superselective sacral nerve resection. *7th ICS Conference*, 67–8.

Heathcote, P. S., Galloway, N. T. M., Lewis, D. C., and Stephenson, T. P. (1987). An assessment of the complications of the Brantley Scott artificial sphincter. *British Journal of Urology*, **60**, 119–21.

Hindmarsh, J. R., Essenhigh, D. M., and Yeates, W. K. (1977). Bladder transection for adult enuresis. *British Journal of Urology*, **49**, 515–21.

Hinman, F. (1976). Post-operative overdistension of the bladder. *Surgery, Gynaecology and Obstetrics*, **142**, 901–2.

Iwatsubo, E., Komine, S., Yamashita, H., Imamura, A., and Akatsu, T. (1984). Overdistension therapy of the bladder in paraplegia patients using self-catheterization. A preliminary study. *Paraplegia*, **22**, 210–15.

Jakobsen, H. and Hald, T. (1986). Management of neurogenic urinary incontinence with AMS artificial urinary sphincter. *Scandinavian Journal of Urology and Nephrology*, **20**, 137–41.

Kato, K., Kondo, A., Takita, T., Gotoh, M., Tanaka, J., and Mitsuya, H. (1987). Incontinence in female neurogenic bladders. Resolution by endoscopic bladder neck suspension. *British Journal of Urology*, **59**, 523–5.

Katona, F. and Eckstein, H. (1974). Treatment of neuropathic bladder by transurethral electrical stimulation. *Lancet*, **i**, 780–1.

Kiely, E. A., Hartnell, G. G., Gibson, R. N., and Williams, G. (1987). Measurement of bladder volume by real-time ultrasound. *British Journal of Urology*, **60**, 33–5.

Kinder, R. B. and Mundy, A. R. (1985). Atropine blockade of nerve-mediated stimulation of the human detrusor. *British Journal of Urology*, **57**, 418–21.

Koyanagi, T., Arikado, K., Takamatsu, T., and Tsuji, I. (1982). Relevance of sympathetic dyssynergia in the region of the external urethral sphincter: possible mechanism of voiding dysfunction in the absence of (somatic) sphincter dyssynergia. *Journal of Urology*, **127**, 277–82.

Koyanagi, T., Takamatsu, T., and Taniguchi, K. (1984). Further characterization of the external urethral sphincter in spinal cord injury: study during spinal shock and evolution of responsiveness to alpha-adrenergic stimulation. *Journal of Urology*, **131**, 1122–6.

Krane, R. and Olsson, C. (1973). Phenoxybenzamine in neurogenic bladder dysfunction II. Clinical considerations. *Journal of Urology*, **110**, 653–6.

Lapides, J., Diokno, A. C., and Silber, S. J. (1972). Clean intermittent self catheterisation in the treatment of urinary tract disease. *Journal of Urology*, **107**, 458–61.

Light, J. K. and Scott, F. B. (1982). Bethanechol chloride and the traumatic cord bladder. *Journal of Urology*, **128**, 85–7.

Light, J. K., Faganel, J., and Beric, A. (1985). Detrusor areflexia in supra sacral cord injuries. *Journal of Urology*, **134**, 295–7.

Lloyd, L. K., Kuhlemeier, K. V., Fine, P. R., and Stover, S. L. (1986). Initial bladder management in spinal cord injury: does it make a difference? *Journal of Urology*, **135**, 523–7.

Low, A. I. and Donovan, W. D. (1981). The use and mechanism of anal sphincter stretch in the reflex bladder. *British Journal of Urology*, **53**, 430–2.

Lucas, M. G. and Thomas, D. G. (1987). Endoscopic bladder transection for detrusor instability. *British Journal of Urology*, **59**, 526–8.

McGuire, E. J. and Savastano, J. A. (1983). Long-term follow up of spinal cord injury patients managed by intermittent catheterisation. *Journal of Urology*, **129**, 775–6.

McGuire, E. J., Morrissey, S., Zhang, S., and Horwinski, E. (1983). Control of reflex detrusor activity in normal and spinal injured non-human primates. *Journal of Urology*, **129**, 197–9.

Malone, P. R., Stanton, S. L., and Riddle, P. R. (1985). Urinary diversion for incontinence—a beneficial procedure? *Annals of the Royal College of Surgeons*, **67**, 349–52.

Mathe, J. F., Labat, J. J., Lanoiselee, J. M., and Buzelin, J. M. (1985). Detrusor inhibition in suprasacral spinal cord injuries: is it due to sympathetic overactivity? *Paraplegia*, **23**, 201–6.

Mathias, C. J. and Frankel, H. L. (1983). Clinical manifestations of malfunctioning sympathetic mechanisms in tetraplegia. *Journal of the Autonomic Nervous System*, **7**, 303–12.

Mobley, D. F. (1976). Phenoxybenzamine in the management of neurogenic vesical dysfunction. *Journal of Urology*, **116**, 737–8.

Moisey, C. U., Stephenson, T. P., and Brendler, C. B. (1980). The urodynamic and subjective results of treatment of detrusor instability with oxybutynin chloride. *British Journal of Urology*, **52**, 472–5.

Montague, D. and Stewart, B. (1979). Urethral pressure profiles before and after ornade administration in patients with stress incontinence. *British Journal of Urology*, **122**, 198–9.

Mundy, A. R. and Stephenson, T. P. (1985). 'Clam' ileocystoplasty for the treatment of refractory urge incontinence. *Journal of Urology*, **57**, 641–6.

Namiki, T., Ito, H., and Yasuda, K. (1978). Management of the urinary tract by suprapubic cystology kept under a closed and aseptic state in the acute stage of the patient with a spinal cord lesion. *Journal of Urology*, **119**, 359–62.

Nicholas, J. L. and Eckstein, H. B. (1975). Endovesical electrotherapy in treatment of urinary incontinence in spina bifida patients. *Lancet*, **ii**, 1276–7.

Nordling, J., Christensen, B., and Gosling, J. L. (1980). Noradrenergic innervation of the human bladder in neurogenic dysfunction. *Urologia Internationalis*, **35**, 188–93.

Nordling, J., Meyhoff, H. H., and Olesen, K. P. (1982). Cysto-urethrographic appearance of the bladder and posterior urethra in neuromuscular disorders of the lower urinary tract. *Scandinavian Journal of Urology and Nephrology*, **16**, 115–24.

O'Flynn, J. D. (1976) An assessment of surgical treatment of vesical outlet obstruction of surgical treatment of vesical outlet obstruction in spinal cord injury: a review of 471 cases. *British Journal of Urology*, **48**, 657–62.

Ott, R. and Rossier, A. B. (1971). L'intérêt du sondage intermittent dans la rééducation vésicale des lésions médullaires traumatique aiguës. *Urologia Internationalis*, **27**, 51–65.

Parsons, K. F., Machin, D. G., Woolfenden, K. A., Walmsley, B., Abercrombie, G. F., and Vinnicombe, J. (1984). Endoscopic bladder transection. *British Journal of Urology*, **56**, 625–8.

Pearman, J. W. (1971). Prevention of urinary tract infection following spinal cord injury. *Paraplegia*, **9**, 95–104.

Pengelly, A. W., Stephenson, T. P., and Milroy, E. J. G. (1978). Results of prolonged bladder distension as treatment for detrusor instability. *British Journal of Urology*, **50**, 243–5.

Perkash, I. and Friedland, G. W. (1986). Transrectal ultrasonography of the lower urinary tract: evaluation of bladder neck problems. *Neurourology and Urodynamics*, **5**, 299–306.

Philp, N. H., Thomas, D. G., and Rickwood, A. M. K. (1983). The effect of anteromedian sphincterotomy on penile erections in patients with neuropathic bladder. *Paraplegia*, **21**, 301–4.

Ross, J. C., Gibbon, N. O. K., and Damanski, M. (1958). Division of the external urethral sphincter in the treatment of the paraplegic bladder. *British Journal of Urology*, **30**, 204–12.

Ruutu, M. L. and Lehtonen, T. A. (1985). Bladder outlet surgery in men with spinal cord injury. *Scandinavian Journal of Urology and Nephrology*, **19**, 241–6.

Schulman, C. C., Simon, J., Wespes, E., and Germeau, F. (1984). Endoscopic injections of teflon to treat urinary incontinence in women. *British Medical Journal*, **288**, 192.

Scott, F. B., Bradley, W. E., and Timm, G. W. (1974). Treatment of urinary incontinence by an implantable prosthetic urinary sphincter. *Journal of Urology*, **112**, 75–80.

Smith, P. H., Cook, J. B., and Rhind, J. R. (1972). Manual expression of the bladder following spinal cord injury. *Paraplegia*, **9**, 213–18.

Stamey, T. A. (1973). Endoscopic suspension of the vesical neck for urinary incontinence. *Surgery, Gynaecology and Obstetrics*, **136**, 547–54.

Tammela, T., Kontturi, M., Kaar, K., and Lukkarinen, O. (1987). Intravesical prostaglandin F_2 alpha for promoting bladder emptying after surgery for female stress incontinence. *British Journal of Urology*, **60**, 43–6.

Thomas, D. G., Smallwood, R., and Graham, D. (1975). Urodynamic observations following spinal trauma. *British Journal of Urology*, **47**, 161–75.

Thomas, D. G., Philp, N. H., McDermott, T. E. D., and Rickwood, A. M. K. (1984).

The use of urodynamic studies to assess the effect of pharmacological agents with particular references to alpha adrenergic blockade. *Paraplegia*, **22**, 162–7.

Torrens, M. J. (1985). The role of denervation in the treatment of detrusor instability. *Neurourology and Urodynamics*, **14**, 353–6.

Vodusek, D. B., Light, J. K., and Libby, J. M. (1986). Detrusor inhibition induced by stimulation of pudendal nerve afferents. *Neurourology and Urodynamics*, **5**, 381–9.

Wein, A. J. (1987). Lower urinary tract function and pharmacologic management of lower urinary tract dysfunction. *Urological Clinics of North America*, **14**, 273–96.

8

Central pain

L. S. Illis

Central pain is the term used for pain, arising from lesions confined to the central nervous system, which is of an intense unbearable nature and often found in association with particularly unpleasant dysaesthesiae. It may be spontaneous or in response to minor stimulation, is usually associated with over-reaction to stimulation, and may be either diffuse or localized. Sensory impairment or loss is invariable. The definition of central pain, however, is not without some ambiguity. Some pain clearly arises from a mixture of peripheral and central causes, for example the pain in arachnoiditis, where peripheral lesions occur and where there is central involvement indicated by the presence of long tract signs. Each year more research indicates that peripheral mechanisms induce central changes, and the division between central and peripheral pain must necessarily become blurred. However, Cline *et al.* (1989) demonstrated, in man, sensitization of C nociceptor receptors with low threshold and prolonged after-discharges (which would explain the abnormal quality of pain and exaggerated response in chronic pain), but with no evidence of secondary CNS dysfunction and no evidence of sympathetic disturbance. There remains, therefore, considerable uncertainty about the mechanisms of both central and peripheral pain.

When pain occurs in spinal lesions most cases show the classical features of central pain: the pain takes time to develop, there is no tissue damage ouside the CNS (as is the case in nociceptive or tissue-damage pain), there is associated sensory deficit, there is the presence of allodynia, i.e. the production of pain by a non-painful stimulus (pathognomonic of neurogenic pain), and there are lower skin temperatures in the painful area, with the frequent exacerbation of pain by temperature changes or emotional stress (suggesting autonomic involvement), and resistance to narcotic analgesia. Spinal cord painful syndromes may be due to vascular lesions or to trauma. In complete lesions, phantom sensation or phantom pain, similar to the description of a phantom limb after amputation, may be referred to any part of the body below the transsection, but is usually referred to the legs or to the feet. In an incomplete lesion such as a Brown–Séquard, the pain is short-lived on the side of the lesion, but may persist for years on the contralateral side. Pain in patients with spinal cord injury is not uncommon, and is dealt with in greater detail by Berić (this volume). Kakulas *et al.* (1990) showed that pain and abnormal sensations are more common in patients with anatomically incomplete injuries, with longer survival, and where there is evidence of regeneration of nerve roots at the level of the lesion.

In spinal cord injury several types of pain may occur. Central pain is usually localized at or below the level of the lesion, and is described as a burning, stabbing, pins and needles type of sensation. That is, the pain is described in terms similar to any other type of central pain. Pain in post-traumatic syringomyelia is localized above the level of the lesion. The pain may begin below the level of paralysis, but always ascends, and is the commonest presenting complaint of post-traumatic syringomyelia. Musculo-skeletal pain usually has an aching quality, is localized at or distal to the lesion, and may be associated with some obvious cause, such as contracture, degenerative joint disease, or fracture. Radicular pain is localized to the lesion site and has a characteristic distribution.

The timing of pain after spinal cord injury is often helpful in diagnosis. Central pain tends to appear earlier (usually within three months), whereas the other pains are usually of much later onset, often after many years.

Pain may occur with non-traumatic syringomyelia, and may precede any other sign of the disease by many years. In multiple sclerosis pain and dysaesthesiae are not unusual, although frequently the patients do not report the pain unless questioned. Lhermitte's sign is usually associated with dis-comfort rather than pain. The localized pain (sometimes of nerve-root distribution) seen with spinal tumours is not strictly pain of central origin. However, painful dysaesthesiae may be referred to areas below the level of the lesion, and in rare cases pain may precede any other symptom or sign. Less common causes of central pain include myelitis and myelopathy secondary to cervical spondylosis.

Parodoxically, surgical lesions designed to alleviate pain, such as cordot-omy and commissural myelotomy, may produce late unpleasant pain which is often quite different from the original pain and is associated with dysaesthesiae.

Suprathalamic lesions may give rise to pain which is similar in its nature to the pain of thalamic syndrome.

Pathophysiology

There is a complex and widespread organization of the nociceptive system ('nociceptive' because it responds to noxious stimuli); but since pain, for most people, is a minor event, the nociceptive system must either be involved in other, and perhaps more important aspects than signalling pain, for example concerned with inflammation or tissue repair, or the system is in almost continuous suppression under normal circumstances. Central pain would then occur if the nociceptive system is 'released', as was suggested by many neurologists and neurophysiologists in the early part of the century. Melzack and Wall's (1965) gate-control theory, which has done so much to stimulate interest and understanding of pain, proposed that nerve-damage interfered with the constant inhibitory modulation of large-diameter fibres and their connections. That is, peripheral activity is coded into a centrally transmitted message in the substantia gelatinosa of the dorsal horn. Centrally evoked excitation is subject to modulation, and changes in this modulation will change the encoded message. Pain afferents may be selectively inhibited at all levels of the central nervous system by both ascending and descending systems via presynaptic inhibition, or by alteration of the excitability of neurons.

Nociceptive mediation involves periventricular and periaqueduct grey matter, the nucleus raphe magnus of the medulla, and the dorsolateral funiculi of the spinal cord, with neurotransmission and modulation via enkephalins and endorphins (the enkephalins- and endorphins-mediating analgesia system: EMAS), and by serotoninergic projections. Electrical stimulation of brainstem structures (Richardson and Akil 1973) and of spinal cord (Krainick and Thoden 1989) partially blocks various clinical syndromes, possibly by activating the EMAS, but may sometimes exacerbate pain following central reorganization following neurological damage (Cole *et al.* 1987).

Partial or total interruption of afferent fibres results in degeneration of appropriate presynaptic terminals and an alteration in function and structure. Denervated synaptic sites may be reinnervated by other axons (i.e sprouting—Liu and Chambers 1958; Illis 1967; Raisman 1969) and previously ineffective synapses may become active (i.e. unmasking—Merrill and Wall 1978). Excitation spreads to neighbouring areas and supersensitivity occurs, producing an abnormal firing pattern which may depend upon stimulation or may occur spontaneously. This sequence of events explains many of the symptoms of central pain, including dysaesthesia (abnormal firing pattern), spontaneous shooting pain (paroxysmal burst discharges), evoked pain from non-painful stimuli, diffusion of the evoked abnormal sensation, and the long-term failure of neurosurgical treatment.

Irritative lesions of sensory pathways possibly produce hypersensitivity, and partial destruction results in the generation of new receptors. However, although this kind of change has been shown to occur in the peripheral nervous system (Wall 1979), it has not been definitely demonstrated in the central nervous system, and central pain may occur even after complete destruction of central sensory pathways. Damage to central sympathetic fibres (cerebro-spinal sensory fibres) possibly produces pain and hyperpathia. Experimental partial lesions of the posterolateral nucleus of the thalamus (Spiegel *et al.* 1954) result in an alteration of the evoked response from the periphery, and although this may explain hyperpathia and dysaesthesiae, it does not explain symptoms in lesions below the thalamus unless partial lesions result in altered transmission characteristics in the spinothalamic and lemniscal systems, so that the central pattern of impulses (spatial and temporal) is abnormal and wrongly interpreted or integrated.

In summary, central pain may be due to abnormal hypersensitivity of damaged fibres, the generation of new receptors, alteration in the central pattern of impulses, alteration of inhibitory mechanisms, including the EMAS, and activation of secondary (polysynaptic) pathways.

The management of central pain

As in all cases of chronic pain the first step is an accurate diagnosis. This involves a careful neurological history and examination, and may also necessitate, in some patients, complex and sophisticated neurophysiological and neuroradiological techniques. Explanation of the diagnosis to the patient and discussion of the nature of intractable pain may have no effect on the severity of the pain, but will make management of the pain much easier from both the doctor's and the sufferer's point of view. This is an essential part of treatment, and continues while drugs, nerve blocks, surgery, and stimulation techniques are applied. All classes of psychotropic drugs, including anti-depressants, neuroleptics,and sedatives have been reported to be beneficial in intractable pain. However, most clinical studies are poorly designed, partly because of the serious problems imposed by the difficulty (or even impossibility) of measuring chronic pain objectively, and partly because of the complex interaction of physical and psychological factors.

Stimulation of central grey matter may produce analgesia, and this has been linked with 5-hydroxytryptamine (5-HT), the neurotransmitter in pathways from the periaqueductal grey matter to the spinal cord. Any manipulation which increases 5-HT is likely to increase analgesia, and any reduction is likely to decrease analgesia. 5-HT probably inhibits nociceptive neurons which project to the spinal cord, and thus reduces pain-transmission. Morphine analgesia is also linked with 5-HT, and destruction of 5-HT pathways blocks the analgesic action of morphine; while stimulation of the dorsal raphe (connected to the periaqueductal grey matter) increases morphine analgesia. Naturally occurring opioids increase after stimulation-produced analgesia. The evidence linking 5-HT, enkephalins, substance P and opioids, and stimulation-produced analgesia is increasing at a rapid rate. In summary, enkephalins and substance P are dorsal horn inhibitory neurotransmitters in the nociceptive pathway which appears to be linked with 5-HT as an ascending and descending tract neurotransmitter. Manipulation of 5-HT alters pain perception. 5-HT is one of the monoamine neurotransmitters (others are noradrenalin and dopamine) linked to the so-called monoamine hypothesis of depression, which proposes that specific features of depression are the result of abnormalities of particular monoamines, and antidepressant action depends on increasing the availability of these amines by producing a specific reuptake inhibition at synaptic level (Walsh 1983).

Use of anti-depressants

The well-known clinical association between chronic pain and depression may have a good pharmacological explanation—namely 5-HT reduction. The use of amitriptyline, regarded as the best antidepressant for its analgesic effect, is supported by pharmacological evidence, since 5-HT appears to be more affected by drugs with a tertiary amine structure. Carbamazepine is a close relative of imipramine, but has no antidepressant effect. Amitriptyline probably acts as a selective synaptic blocker of 5-HT synaptic reuptake, but also ameliorates psychological stress and produces non-specific depression of arousal, and thus may modify the central perception of pain. Intractable pain is associated with changes in personality which regress with effective pain-treatment, and it is perhaps necessary to document personality disturbance only as it affects the complaint of intractable pain, rather than attempt to implicate such disturbance in the aetiology of the pain. About 60 per cent of patients with chronic illness also suffer from depression (Walsh 1983). Conversely, pain is common in depressive illness. Depression and anxiety are influenced by insight, perception, and by the doctor's own perception of pain, and these factors must be included in the general management of chronic intractable pain.

Use of anti-convulsants

The use of anticonvulsant drugs in intractable pain stems from the original trial of phenytoin in trigeminal neuralgia (Bergouignan 1942). Carbamazepine was introduced in 1962 (Blom 1962), and since then anticonvulsant drugs have been used for a variety of paroxysmal lancinating pains and for central pain. The mode of action is uncertain, but the anticonvulsant property is probably not relevant, since anti-epileptic barbiturate drugs have no effect in chronic pain. Phenytoin appears to stabilize hyperexcitability caused by low calcium levels, and blocks post-tetanic potentiation. Carbamazepine also depresses post-tetanic potentiation and inhibits polysynaptic reflex activity (Theobald et al. 1970). Anticonvulsants may affect the high-frequency discharge characteristic of ectopic pace-makers—that is, the anomalous repetitive firing of axons seen after injury, demyelination, metabolic disturbance, or ischaemia. Yaari and Devor (1985) showed that phenytoin may block such discharges without blocking nerve-conduction, so that the analgesic effect may be peripheral rather than central.

Use of nerve blocks

Peripheral nerve blocks, including section of nerve roots, have been attempted for treatment of pain, and the results are inconsistent. An anaesthetic block is worth attempting, since temporary relief may occur. Nerve blocks serve a diagnostic as well as a therapeutic use, since pain-relief following a specific block implies that the painful stimuli arose from the site anaesthetized. However, the perception of pain depends on the reception of specific signals at cerebral level. The source of these signals is deduced from previous patterns. Pain, therefore, can occur or be perceived when signals are initiated within the central nervous system and without any peripheral tissue damage, or after the initial peripheral damage has healed.

The interpretation of the response to nerve block is not always straight-forward. For example, pain-relief from nerve block (short-term) is not always an accurate predictor for surgical destructive techniques (Loeser 1972). Nor can nerve blocks (for example, epidural) separate peripheral from central origin, since the local anaesthetic may be locally absorbed, or may alter sensory input.

The therapeutic use of nerve blocks include pain prevention. For example, epidural block carried out some days before amputation may reduce the frequency and severity of phantom-limb pain (Bach *et al.* 1988). In pain where there is a sympathetic efferent component (reflex sympathetic dystrophy, sympathetically maintained pain) diagnostic sympathetic blocks will elucidate the degree of contribution. One of the major indications for nerve blockade is in reflex sympathetic dystrophy or sympathetically main-tained pain.

Sympathetic block reduces the effect of sympathetic modulation on receptors, and may be of short-lived benefit (Loh *et al.* 1982). Depletion of noradrenalin in postganglionic sympathetic terminals by guanethidine block (Hannington-Kiff 1974) may be effective.

Use of surgical techniques

Neurosurgical operations, including cordotomy and tractotomies, resection of sensory cortex, and stereotactic operations at thalamic level, are generally disappointing, as indicated earlier. Neurosurgical treatment of chronic pain was based on a fairly rigid interpretation of anatomy. This destruction approach or disconnection of various pathways has now largely given way to methods which alter or influence sensory input and are based on the inter-pretation of experimental anatomical and physiological work. Although neurosurgical (ablative) procedures have been used for many years, there are obvious limitations to these procedures. Total denervation of a painful area would usually be impossible, selective destruction of nociceptive fibres cannot be guaranteed, and the anatomy is rarely straightforward: for example the presence of afferent C fibres within ventral roots.

Dorsal root entry zone lesions (DREZ) may be effective in pain, but micro-surgical DREZ lesions which aim to destroy facilitatory pathways are probably more effective (Sindou and Jeanmond 1990).

Ascending pain pathways in the spinal cord may be interrupted by commisural myelotomy (section of midline decussation) or by anterolateral cordotomy (section of contralateral ascending projection). Unilateral cordotomy may be insufficient, since not all fibres decussate at spinal level, and ipsilateral pain may appear post-operatively. Bilateral cordotomy may result in permanent disturbances of blood-pressure and sphincter control. There is no neurosurgical ablative technique for pain without neurological side-effects which are normally unacceptable.

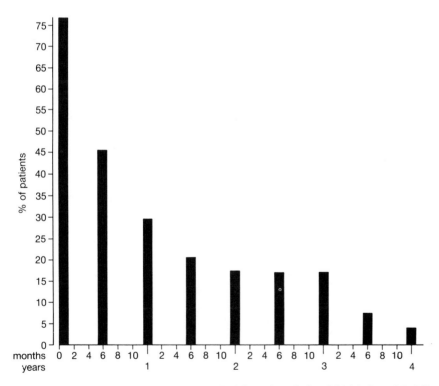

Fig. 8.1. Percentage of patients with worthwhile pain relief (+3/+4/+5 on McGill pain score), over four years. The data is from 39 patients (conditions indicated in Table 8.1).

Table 8.1. Pain—response to spinal cord stimulation (numbers refer to alteration in McGill pain score)

−1	0	+2	+3	+4	+5
Arachnoiditis	Spinal injury	Multiple sclerosis	Multiple sclerosis	Multiple sclerosis	Reflex sympathetic dystrophy
	Spinal injury	Peripheral vascular disease	Multiple sclerosis	Multiple sclerosis	Peripheral vascular disease
	Spinal injury	Peripheral vascular disease	Arachnoiditis	Multiple sclerosis	
	Spinal injury		Arachnoiditis	Multiple sclerosis	
	Spinal A/V malformation		Syphilitic transverse myelitis	Multiple sclerosis	
	Phantom pain		Arachnoiditis	Multiple sclerosis	
	Peripheral vascular disease		Fractured rib	Peripheral vascular disease	
	Peripheral vascular disease		Arachnoiditis	Peripheral vascular disease	
	Peripheral vascular disease		Peripheral vascular disease	Arachnoiditis	
				Phantom pain	
				Radiation myelitis	
				Diabetic polyneuritis	
				Ischemic cord lesion	
				Peripheral vascular disease	
				Peripheral vascular disease	

Use of stimulation

Electrical stimulation has been carried out ever since Melzack and Wall's original description of 'gate-control'. Spinal cord and peripheral stimulation techniques have, as their basis, the rationale of enhancing the inhibitory function of primary afferents. Peripheral nerve stimulation, often effective in pain of peripheral origin, is not usually effective in central pain. Spinal cord stimulation may be extremely effective in some patients, and the results are longer-lasting and cause no disability compared to neurosurgical procedures (Illis *et al.* 1983; Koeze *et al.* 1987); but it is unlikely to help in pain due to spinal cord injury (Cole *et al.* 1991). The results of 39 patients with intractable pain treated with spinal cord stimulation are summarized in Table 8.1. Figure 8.1 indicates the pain-relief obtained with spinal cord stimulation. Although there is a very good initial result, the mean duration of response is 1 year 6 months. Intracerebral stimulation (deep-brain stimulation) is still considered a somewhat uncertain method of treatment, because of the great variability in reported results, and this is discussed in detail by Gybels *et al.* (1990).

In conclusion, the management of central pain is by no means a settled question, but nor should it be considered a field of therapeutic nihilism. A great deal can be done to help the patient provided a methodical approach is taken and neurosurgical procedures are only considered as a last resort.

(This chapter is based on Illis, L. S. (1990). Central pain, *British Medical Journal*, **300**, 1284–86.)

References

Bach, S., Noreng, M. F., and Tjellden, N. U. (1988). Phantom limit pain in amputees during the first 12 months following limb amputation after pre-operative lumbar epidural blockade. *Pain* **33**, 297–301.

Bergouignan, M. (1942). Cures heureuses de neuralgies faciales essentialles par le diphenyl-hydentoinate de soude. *Revue de Laryngologie, Otologie et Rhinologie*, **63**, 34–41.

Blom, S. (1962). Trigeminal neuralgia: its treatment with a new anti-convulsant drug (G. 32883). *Lancet*, **i**, 839–40.

Cline, M. A., Ochoa, J., and Torebjork, H. E. (1989). Chronic hyperalgesia and skin warming caused by sensitized C nociceptors. *Brain*, **112**, 621–47.

Cole, J. D., Illis, L. S., and Sedgwick, E. M. (1987). Pain produced by spinal cord stimulation in a patient with allodynia and pseudo-tabes. *Journal of Neurology, Neurosurgery and Psychiatry*, **50**, 1083–4.

Cole, J. D., Illis, L. S., and Sedgwick, E. M. (1991). Intractable pain in spinal cord injury is not relieved by spinal cord stimulation. *Paraplegia*, **29**, 167–72.

Gybels, J., Kupers, R., and van Calenbergh (1990). Physiological approach to management of pain. *Recent achievements in restorative neurology, 3: Altered sensation and pain* (ed. M. R. Dimitrijevic, P. D. Wall, and U. Lindblom), pp. 79–86. Karger, Basle.

Hannington-Kiff, J. G. (1974). Intravenous regional sympathetic block with guanethidine. *Lancet*, **i**, 1019–20.

Illis, L. S. (1967) The motoneurone surface and spinal shock. In *Modern trends in neurology*, 4 (ed. D. Williams), pp. 53–8. Butterworth, Sevenoaks.

Illis, L. S., Read, D. J., Sedgwick, E. M., and Tallis, R. C. (1983). Spinal cord stimulation in the United Kingdom. *Journal of Neurology, Neurosurgery, and Psychiatry*, **46**, 299–304.

Kakulas, B. A., Smith, E., Gaekwad, V., Kaelan, C., and Jacobsen, P. F. (1990). The neuropathology of pain and abnormal sensations in human spinal cord injury derived from the clinicopathological data base at the Royal Perth Hospital. In *Recent advances in restorative neurology, 3. Altered sensation of pain* (ed. M. R. Dimitrijevic, P. D. Wall, and U. Lindblom), pp. 37–41. Karger, Basle.

Koeze, T. H., Williams, A. C. de C., and Reiman, S. (1987). Spinal cord stimulation and the relief of chronic pain. *Journal of Neurology, Neurosurgery, and Psychiatry*, **50**, 1424–9.

Krainick, J-U. and Thoden, U. (1989). Spinal cord stimulation. In *Textbook of pain* (ed. P. D. Wall and R. Melzack), Chapter 66, pp. 920–4. Churchill Livingstone, Edinburgh.

Liu, G. N. and Chambers, W. W. (1958). Intraspinal sprouting of dorsal root axons. *Archives of Neurology and Psychiatry (Chicago)*, **79**, 46–61.

Loeser, J. D. (1972). Dorsal rhizotomy for the relief of chronic pain. *Journal of Neurosurgery*, **36**, 745–50.

Loh, L., Nathan, P. W., and Schott, G. D. (1982). Pain due to lesions of the central nervous system removed by sympathetic block. *British Medical Journal*, **282**, 1026–8.

Melzack, R. and Wall, P. D. (1965). Pain mechanisms: a new theory. *Science*, **150**, 971–9.

Merrill, E. G. and Wall, P. D. (1978). Plasticity of connections in the adult nervous system. In *Neuronal plasticity* (ed. C. W. Cotman), pp. 97–111. Raven Press, New York.

Raisman, G. (1969). Neuronal plasticity in the septal nuclei of the adult rat. *Brain Research*, **14**, 25–48.

Richardson, D. E. and Akil, H. (1973). Pain relief by electrical stimulation of the brain in human patients. *Excerpta Medica*, **393**, 79.

Sindou, M. and Jeanmond, D. (1990). Structural approach to the management of pain. In *Recent achievements in restorative neurology, 3: Altered sensation and pain* (ed. M. R. Dimitrijević, P. D. Wall, and U. Lindblom), pp. 64–78. Karger, Basle.

Spiegel, E. A., Kletzkin, M., Szekely, E. G., and Wycis, H. T. (1954). Role of hypothalamic mechanisms in thalamic pain. *Neurology*, **4**, 739–51.

Theobald, W., Krupp, P., and Levin, P. (1970). Neuropharmacologic aspects of the therapeutic action of carbamazepine on trigeminal neuralgia. In *Trigeminal neuralgia pathogenesis and pathophysiology* (ed. R. Hassler and A. E. Walker), pp. 107–14. Geo. Thieme, Stuttgart.

Wall, P. D. (1979). Changes in damaged nerve and their sensory consequences. In *Advances in pain research and therapy, 3* (ed. J. J. Bonica, J. C. Liebeskind, and D. Albe-Fessard), pp. 205–231. Raven Press, New York.

Walsh, T. D. (1983). Antidepressants in chronic pain. *Clinical Neuropharmacology*, **6**, 271–95.

Yaari, Y. and Devor, M. (1985). Phenytoin suppresses spontaneous ectopic discharge in rat sciatic neuromas. *Neuroscience Letters*, **58**, 117–22.

9

Pain in spinal cord injury

Aleksandar Berić

Sustaining a spinal cord injury (SCI), even a severe one, does not necessarily entail pain, although a majority of SCI patients in the acute phase do experience pain, which usually subsides with medical management. In the chronic phase, however, about one-third of SCI patients complain of sensory disturbances, either pain or unpleasant sensations called dysaesthesiae. In chronic SCI patients it is not only the incidence of pain, but its intractability which is important. In these patients we are dealing with two problems: one is the chronic pain syndrome, with all its complexities; and the other is a chronic neurogenic dysfunction with a poorly understood pathophysiology. In treating pain there are additional complicating factors: the patients' ages, their need for rehabilitation, and the limited availability of drugs which do not interfere with cognitive functions and memory. Once their condition is stable patients may have a normal life expectancy, and, as the underlying neurological dysfunction will continue, the pain may also remain. Therefore the need for treatment of chronic pain continues for years, and the potential for developing drug-tolerance and addiction must be addressed prior to the onset of therapy. Before reviewing treatment and intervention for pain in SCI, some of the most important problems in establishing the presence of pain and its possible causes will be discussed, as well as the importance of reported studies on pain-management in SCI. There are several extensive reviews of the topic (Burke and Woodward 1976; Bedbrook 1981). A recent review by Tunks (1986) covered in detail the majority of pertinent reported studies of pain in SCI. This chapter will concentrate upon neurogenic pain in SCI, particularly pain which might have been caused by injury to the spinal cord.

Incidence and onset of pain

The incidence of pain from the acute and on through the chronic stage of SCI varies with the individual course of recovery and the appearance of complications. Injuries at the cervical level are especially difficult to assess, as the patients tend to have more respiratory complications. If the injury is more severe, requiring spine stabilization with a variable period of immobilization, or includes head injury, the result is a prolonged hospital course. These patients often have urinary tract infections, severe postural hypotension, and irregular bowel function, which all further extend the acute period. As pain is a subjective experience, it is also influenced by patients' separation from the community and family, as well as by psychological difficulties related to their disability, changes in life-style, and financial matters. These are all issues which must be considered in the early assessment of pain.

It would be advantageous to understand the underlying cause of pain in acute SCI patients, because the outcome depends on the origin. For instance, early burning pain, early 'end zone' pain (Burke and Woodward 1976), and pain due to soft tissue and skeletal injury of the nociceptive type all have a tendency to improve with time and after general management of acute injury. The major problem seems to be the distinction between pain related to spinal cord and cauda equina injury and injury to other tissues, such as musculo-skeletal injuries or concomitant nerve and plexus injuries. Strictly speaking, these are not SCI pains but SCI-related pains, which become almost inseparable in cases such as cervical SCI and concomitant brachial plexus injury.

This leads us to the chronic stage, where the same problem of separation of the cause and the type of pain exists. As these patients usually have decreased sensory perception below the level of the lesion, visceral pains due to infections, calculi, or late spinal instability may be inappropriately included as genuine spinal cord pain. Another distinction to be made is between the pain related to the initial spinal injury, and pain related to its complications, such as post-traumatic syringomyelia. This is obviously an unsettled issue, which, without knowledge of the underlying pathology and pathophysiology, is probably better left alone. When all the difficulties are considered, it is not surprising to find the reported incidence of pain in SCI ranging from 10 to 90 per cent (Munro 1950; Botterell *et al.* 1953; Krueger 1960). Our own figures show that in a population of more severe SCIs the incidence of neurogenic SCI pain appears to be about 50 per cent (Berić 1990). Investigating the incidence of chronic pain in SCI patients, using a postal questionnaire, Rose *et al.* (1988) considered not only pain perception, but also the effects of pain on activity. In a sample of 885 patients, 98 said that pain and not paralysis stopped them working, 325 said pain interfered with sleep, and 118 reported that pain could be severe enough to stop social activity.

Pain or dysaesthesia?

Another important problem in assessment of pain in SCI is the presence of spontaneous sensations such as paraesthesiae, which usually do not require treatment and most of the time are well tolerated. However, the intensity of such sensations may fluctuate, and patients might want to know the cause of this fluctuation in a follow-up visit. It is usually relatively easy to resolve the problem by comparison with the previous status. Dysaesthesiae, on the other hand, are usually more diffuse, quite often functionally limiting, and in most cases will require treatment (Davis and Martin 1947; Davis 1975; Davidoff *et al.* 1987; Berić *et al.* 1988). The distinctions between pain, dysaesthesiae, and paraesthesiae are subjective; but there is an important qualitative difference. In patients with a clinically complete absence of sensory and motor functions below the level of lesion all these phenomena are sometimes combined with phantom sensations (Guttmann 1976), or even called phantom pain (Melzack and Loeser 1978), a term based on our poor understanding of the pathophysiology.

Description of pain and classification

As pain is a subjective experience, we have to describe its distribution, intensity, and quality precisely. Distribution is obtainable from a pain-drawing by the patient. Intensity is assessed from visual analogue scales which are labelled with respect to the sensory experience. In addition, separate categorical scales from 0 to 5 for emotional and function-limiting intensity might be used. Finally, quality is assessed, both open-endedly, being completely open to the patient's description, and also with a list of different qualities of pain, dysaesthesiae, and paraesthesiae; such as aching, burning, pins and needles, throbbing, etc. Often the McGill Pain Questionnaire is used (Melzack 1975), although it should be modified for SCI patients. Patients find some of the offered groups offensive, and often the full variety of their dysaesthetic complaints is not covered. We usually combine topography with quality, by offering the patient various patterns for the different qualities to fill into the pain-drawing. These two instruments, pain-drawings including topography and quality and visual analogue scales, are obtainable in a very short period of time, and can be used both for short-term follow-up, i.e. during and after the temporary nerve blocks, or in long-term follow-up with or without treatment. Further distinctions for both pain and dysaesthesiae can be made (a) relative to distribution as superficial or deep distribution, and (b) relative to localization, either as precise or imprecise and with or without clear borders. Pain can be spontaneous, ongoing, or evoked, triggered by any kind of stimulation. Also, it is important to know if it is oligosegmental, covering one or two spinal segments, or is plurisegmental or diffuse.

Any classifications based on presumptive underlying mechanisms are difficult to apply in individual cases without scientific testing of the proposed mechanisms. For practical purposes, a descriptive and phenomenological approach might be more appropriate (Davis 1975; Burke and Woodward 1976).

Clinical and neurophysiological assessment

In the clinical setting, major sensory modalities are usually tested quantitatively for changes in thresholds. Qualitative changes and altered sensation phenomena (Lindblom 1985) are usually inconsistently tested and pursued only if mentioned by patients. Most of the evoked phenomena are usually found in the transitional zone, and almost never below the level of lesion, certainly in patients with complete absence of sensory perception below the level of lesion. Exceptionally, we have had several patients who did have some hypersensitivity and altered qualitative phenomena, usually well localized, below the level of almost complete lesions. One of the patients turned out to have sciatica with a typical root irritation supported by radiological findings, and other patients had entrapment neuropathy of the iliohypogastric nerve. Therefore it is important to take note of these phenomena, as they usually suggest a focal peripheral nerve or root lesion unrelated to the primary spinal cord injury, and are usually treatable.

Clinical assessment should include the distribution of quantitative changes in sensory perception for the major modalities of sensation. There are two major ascending systems, one being anterolateral, responsible for perception of temperature and pain, and the other, the dorsal column-medial lemniscus system (DC-ML) for light touch perception, vibratory perception, proprioception, joint position, and discriminative sensation. As has been shown in incomplete patients, only some of these modalities are abnormal, and in almost complete patients only some of these modalities are partially preserved (Berić et al. 1987a). Thus, it is necessary to test at least two or three modalities of each system, as described in the report by Berić (1989). We test cold and warm perception using heated and cooled metal rollers, with mapping of the sensory abnormalities. Hot and cold pain perception is tested in several discrete areas, including the hands, the feet, and at the level of the lesion. For the DC-ML system we test touch perception over the entire body. In addition semiquantitative von Frey testing is done at least over the hands and feet. Vibratory sensibility is tested quantitatively over the hands, feet, and lower legs with a vibrameter. Joint-position sense and proprioception is tested and measured at major arm and leg joints and index-finger, little-finger, and great-toe joints. We also test graphaesthesia or simple vertical and horizontal line perception, at least over the ball of the index finger and the dorsum of the foot.

In addition, several neurophysiological techniques are used to find additional neurogenic abnormalities. The presence of significant lower motor neuron lesions of lumbo-sacral segments in patients with cervical spinal cord injury would indicate a double lesion which can be easily documented on the basis of abnormality of the LSEPs, by abnormality of bladder function, and by appropriate radiological studies (Berić et al. 1987b; Berić and Light 1988). On the other hand, normal LSEPs, tendon jerks, plantar reflex, and no significant lower motor neuron dysfunction in patients with diffuse dysaesthesiae would exclude peripheral nervous system dysfunction as an explanation for their problem and more firmly label them as a central dysaesthesia syndrome (Berić *et al.* 1988).

These are the questions posed in SCI patients:

1. What is the state of the cord below the level of the lesion?
2. Is there a concomitant peripheral nerve or root lesion?
3. Is there a double spinal cord lesion or occult cauda equina lesion?
4. Is there any dysfunction above the level of lesion.

Certain syndromes can be described on the basis of patients' descriptions, clinical neurological findings, and neurophysiological findings on the peripheral nerve and spinal cord below the level of lesion. In addition, the effect of blocks and techniques such as transcutaneous nerve stimulation (TENS) and spinal cord stimulation (SCS), and medications such as amitriptyline, carbamazepine, clonidine, etc., for the pain or dysaesthesiae, should always be assessed and reported.

Treatment

The major problem in comparing different techniques in the treatment of pain in SCI is the inconsistency in assessment and terminology (Richardson *et al.* 1980; Nashold and Bullitt 1981; Glynn *et al.* 1986). Some reports combine spinal cord and cauda equina injuries (Davis and Martin 1947; Krueger 1960; Druckman and Lende 1965; Richter and Seitz 1984). Some reports combine different types of pain, such as transition zone pain together with diffuse pain (Kaplan *et al.* 1962), or do not specify the type of pain at all (Wycis and Spiegel 1962).

The majority of the reports are case-studies. Some of them contain elaborate discussions of the causes of pain and the results of treatment on the basis of an isolated case (Druckman and Lende 1965). Even when several cases of pain were reported, they had different distributions and qualities of pain (Botterell *et al.* 1953), or several different preceding procedures (Nashold and Bullitt 1981). Sometimes traumatic and non-traumatic cases of spinal cord dysfunction were combined (Kaplan *et al.* 1962; Wycis and Spiegel 1962; Cain 1965). Surprisingly the majority of the cases in the available literature were of cauda equina or lower thoraco-lumbar injuries (Davis and Martin 1947; Botterell *et al.* 1953; Melzack and Loeser 1978; Nashold and Bullitt 1981), and seldom were cases with cervical or high thoracic level reported. This would probably indicate the poor outcome of cervical spinal cord injuries in the 40s, 50s, and 60s, (Munroe 1950); but as the number of surviving cervical spinal cord injury patients increases, especially high quadriplegics, we see more and more pain and dysaesthesia cases with high-level injuries. Our major effort has been to describe different syndromes accompanied with pain and dysaesthesia in high spinal cord injuries (Berić *et al.* 1987*b*, 1988). When trying to find effective treatment modalities for these patients we concluded that there are no studies to prove or disprove the effectiveness of any of the treatment modalities in this patient population, as was also concluded in the thorough review by Tunks (1986). The only recent, adequate study is by Davidoff *et al.* (1987), assessing the effect of trazodone (antidepressant) in the treatment of SCI patients with dysaesthesiae, unfortunately with negative results.

In general, management of neurogenic pain in SCI is by systemic or local pharmacology and by neuro-augmentative and neuro-destructive interventions. Without better insight into underlying mechanisms of pain in SCI, the general management strategies are practically the same as in any other type of pain. Some recent reviews covered the present state of the available techniques, in particular a monograph by Fields (1987).

Pharmacological approach

The pharmacological approach covers non-steroidal analgesics, opioids, antidepressants and anticonvulsants (Bedbrook 1981; Tunks 1986). Owing to the chronic nature of pain, long-term opioid therapy is not desirable, while antidepressants have increased in popularity because of their additional pain-relieving effect in lower dosages. Also anti-epileptics such as phenytoin and carbamazepine, suggested by their effectiveness in trigeminal neuralgia, were tried in SCI patients with chronic pain (Davis 1975). No controlled studies have been published on the effect of these drugs in a well-defined traumatic SCI population except for the negative results with trazodone in dysaesthesia (Davidoff *et al.* 1987). Glynn *et al.* (1986) published an interesting study on the effect of opioid and noradrenergic systems on pain in SCI. They suggested that there may be an independent effect of the drugs which act on these two systems.

Neuro-augmentative procedures

Neuro-augmentative procedures are based on physiological mechanisms and preservation of the input to the nervous system, and can be divided into peripheral nerve stimulation, such as TENS, epidural spinal stimulation (SCS), and central thalamic stimulation. The effects of any such stimulation could be explained by the general principles of the gate-control theory of pain (Melzack and Wall 1965; Wall 1978). As in the majority of the patients there is severe interruption of the ascending systems, with a concomitant diminution or abolition of the large fibre input, effectiveness of TENS and SCS is expected to be definitely reduced. Reports in SCI patients support this speculation (Richardson *et al.* 1980). However, in transitional zone pain (Davis and Lentini 1975) and in some more incomplete patients, these might be helpful, as the situation is similar or identical to that of the peripheral nervous system injuries. Thalamic stimulation, on the other hand, has not been fully explored in spinal cord injury patients.

We have reported negative results of SCS in SCI patients with dysaesthesia (Berić *et al.* 1988). Cole *et al.* 1991 has similar preliminary results using spinal cord stimulation for chronic pain in SCI patients. In fact, the stimulation increased the intensity of dysaesthesiae and supported very different underlying mechanisms of dysaesthesiae in comparison to pain. These findings are in accordance with post-operative assessment of sensory complaints in patients undergoing neurosurgical ablative procedures, where it was shown that in patients with interruption of the spinothalamic system and preservation of the dorsal column system there is high incidence of dysaesthesiae (Pagni 1979). We believe, therefore, that any procedure which increases the disproportion between spinothalamic and dorsal column systems will worsen the situation and is not desirable, regardless of whether it is dorsal column stimulation or interruption of the spinothalamic system by high thoracic or cervical anterolateral cordotomy, mesencephalic tractotomy, or commissural myelotomy.

Neuro-destructive procedures

Neuro-destructive procedures can be directed toward peripheral nerves, spinal cord, brainstem, or thalamus, and can even include pre-frontal lobotomy. These procedures can be chemical, with substances such as phenol in different concentrations, or alcohol. The special case is a use of local anaesthetics for short-term effects and assessment. The neurosurgical techniques are the same regardless of whether they are employed for SCI pain, cancer pain, or other types of pain. There are several excellent neurosurgical reviews which cover the subject (White and Sweet 1969; Maspes and Pagni 1974; Pagni 1979; Sindou and Daher 1988). Neuro-destructive procedures may be grouped differently. For example, according to the specificity or lack of specificity with respect to the pain ascending system. They can be performed at different levels of neural axis. Non-specific deafferentation procedures include neurectomies, rhizotomies, and myelotomies. The procedures which concentrate on interruption of ascending pain systems are commissural myelotomy, anterolateral cordotomy, and medullary and mesencephalic tractotomy, as well as thalamotomy (Davis and Martin 1947; Munro 1950; Botterell *et al.* 1953; Bedbrook 1981; Wycis and Spiegel 1962; Porter *et al.* 1966). Dorsal root entry zone (DREZ) surgery is a special case in the specific group, consisting of destruction of cells in the dorsal horn of the cord that may generate and transmit exaggerated responses rostrally (Sindou *et al.* 1974; Nashold and Bullitt 1981; Nashold 1984; Richter and Seitz 1984).

Conclusion

In conclusion, it is important to identify the underlying cause of pain in every patient with SCI, because if it is nociceptive acute pain, or chronic non-neurogenic pain, it should be treated according to the general guidelines for such pains (Burke and Woodward 1976). If it is chronic neurogenic pain, we should determine if there is any peripheral nerve or root dysfunction which might be responsible for triggering pain, and then try to correct or eliminate the cause. If this is impossible, then interruption of the pain ascending system might be feasible, but the chance of developing dysaesthesias or worsening the existing dysaesthesiae is highly probable, and as we do not have any good specific medication or other procedure for treating dysaesthesiae, the outcome might be worse than the initial problem. We believe that the distinction between pain and dysaesthesiae is important, and should be sought by quantitative sensory testing and neurophysiological assessment. If our hypothesis is correct, pain and dysaesthesiae represent very different categories of neurogenic dysfunction. That is the reason why we do not favour neuroablative procedures in SCI patients for dysaesthesiae or even in those cases where we can identify the peripheral triggering mechanism for pain. If we can, on the other hand, identify the DREZ as hyperactive and possibly responsible for triggering and maintaining the pain, then the DREZ operation is desirable.

Overall, the management of intractable pain in SCI patients should begin with clinical, psychological, and neurophysiological assessments, and, if necessary, other ancillary procedures, such as X-rays, CT, and MRI, in an attempt to establish the intensity and functionally limiting characteristics of pain as well as possibly treatable underlying causes. The next step is controlled trials with antidepressants, anti-epileptics, and neuro-augmentative procedures such as peripheral nerve or spinal cord stimulation. If none of these approaches are satisfactory we would favour DREZ surgery for cauda equina and conus lesions, and remain open to the possibility of better defined neuro-augmentative procedures (Bedbrook 1981), particularly at higher levels such as the thalamus or internal capsule for other patients.

Acknowledgements

Thanks are due to Miss Debra Burt and Mrs Helen Spencer for secretarial assistance. Supported by the Vivian L. Smith Foundation for Restorative Neurology, Houston, Texas.

References

Bedbrook, G. M. (1981). *The care and management of spinal cord injuries*, pp. 224–9. Springer-Verlag, New York.

Berić, A. (1989). Quantitative techniques in assessment of sensory abnormalities in patients with spinal cord injury. In *Quantifying neurologic performance* (ed. R. Davis *et al.*), pp. 84–95. Hanley and Belfus, Inc., Philadelphia.

Berić, A. (1990). Altered sensation and pain in spinal cord injury. In *Recent achievements in restorative neurology*, Vol. 3 (ed. M. R. Dimitrijević, P. D. Wall, and U. Lindblom), pp. 27–36. S. Karger, Basle.

Berić, A. and Light, K. (1988). Correlation of bladder dysfunction and LSEP S wave abnormality in spinal cord injured patients. *Neurology and Urodynamics*, **7**, 131–40.

Berić, A., Dimitrijević, M. R. and Lindblom, U. (1987*a*) Cortical evoked potentials and somatosensory perception in chronic spinal cord injury patients. *Journal of Neurological Science*, **80**, 333–42.

Berić, A., Dimitrijević, M. R., and Light, J. K. (1987*b*). A clinical syndrome of rostral and caudal spinal injury: neurological, neurophysiological and urodynamic evidence for occult sacral lesion. *Journal of Neurology, Neurosurgery and Psychiatry*, **50**, 600–6.

Berić, A., Dimitrijević, M. R., and Lindblom, U. (1988). Central dysesthesia syndrome in spinal cord injury patients. *Pain*, **34**, 109–16.

Botterell, E. H., Callaghan, J. C., and Jousse, A. T. (1953). Pain in paraplegia. Clinical management and surgical treatment. *Proceedings of the Royal Society of Medicine*, **47**, 17–24.

Burke, D. C. and Woodward, J. M. (1976). Injuries of the spine and spinal cord. Part II. In *Handbook of clinical neurology*, Vol. 26 (ed. P. J. Vinken and G. W. Bruyn), pp. 489–99. North-Holland, Amsterdam.

Cain, H. D. (1965). Subarachnoid phenol block in the treatment of pain and spasticity. *Paraplegia*, **3**, 152–60.

Cole, J. D., Illis, L. S., and Sedgwick, E. N. (1991) Intractable pain in spinal cord injury is not relieved by spinal cord stimulation. *Paraplegia*, **29**, 167–72.

Davidoff, G., Guarracini, M., Roth, E., Sliwa, J., and Yarkony, G. (1987). Trazodone hydrochloride in the treatment of dysesthetic pain in traumatic myelopathy: a randomized, double-blind, placebo-controlled study. *Pain*, **29**, 151–61.

Davis, L. and Martin, J. (1947). Studies upon spinal cord injuries. II. The nature and treatment of pain. *Archives of Surgery*, **4**, 483–91.

Davis, R. (1975). Pain and suffering following spinal cord injury. *Clinics in Orthopaedics and Related Research*, **112**, 76–80.

Davis, R. and Lentini, R. (1975). Transcutaneous nerve stimulation for treatment of pain in patients with spinal cord injury. *Surgical Neurology*, **4**, 100–1.

Druckman, R. and Lende, R. (1965). Central pain of spinal cord origin. Pathogenesis and surgical relief in one patient. *Neurology*, **15**, 518–22.

Fields, H. L. (1987). *Pain*, pp. 251–334. McGraw-Hill, New York.

Glynn, C. I., Teddy, P. J., Jamous, M. A., Moore, R. A., and Lloyd, J. W. (1986). Role of spinal noradrenergic system in transmission of pain in patients with spinal cord injury. *Lancet*, **2**(8518), 1249–50.

Guttmann, L. (1976). *Spinal cord injuries*, pp. 280–94. Blackwell Scientific, Oxford.

Kaplan, L. I., Grynbaum, B. B., Lloyd, K. E., and Rusk, H. A. (1962). Pain and spasticity in patients with spinal cord dysfunction. Results of a follow-up study. *Journal of the American Medical Association*, **182**, 918–25.

Krueger, E. G. (1960). Management of painful states in injuries of the spinal cord and cauda equina. *American Journal of Physical Medicine*, **39**, 103–10.

Lindblom, U. (1985). Assessment of abnormal evoked pain in neurological patients and its relation to spontaneous pain: a descriptive and conceptual model with some analytical results. In *Advances in pain research and therapy*, Vol. 9 (ed. H. L. Fields *et al.*), pp. 409–23. Raven Press, New York.

Maspes, P. E. and Pagni, C. A. (1974). A critical appraisal of pain surgery and suggestions for improving treatment. In *Recent advances on pain. Pathophysiology and clinical aspects* (ed. J. J. Bonica *et al.*), pp. 201–55. Charles C. Thomas, Springfield, IL.

Melzack, R. (1975). The McGill pain questionnaire: major properties and scoring methods. *Pain*, **1**, 277–99.

Melzack, R. and Loeser, J. D. (1978). Phantom body pain in paraplegics: evidence for a central 'pattern generating mechanism' for pain. *Pain*, **4**, 195–210.

Melzack, R. and Wall, P. D. (1965). Pain mechanisms: a new theory. *Science*, **150**, 971–9.

Munro, D. (1950). Two-year end-results in the total rehabilitation of veterans with spinal-cord and cauda-equina injuries. *New England Journal of Medicine*, **242**, 1–16.

Nashold, B. S. (1984). Current status of the DREZ operation: 1984. *Neurosurgery*, **15**, 942–4.

Nashold, B. S. and Bullitt, E. (1981). Dorsal root entry zone lesions to control central pain in paraplegics. *Journal of Neurosurgery*, **55**, 414–19.

Pagni, C. A. (1976). Central pain and painful anesthesia. *Progress in Neurological Surgery*, **8**, 132–257.

Pagni, C. A. (1979). General comments on ablative neurosurgical procedures. In *Advances in pain research and therapy*, Vol. 2 (ed. J. J. Bonica and V. Ventafridda), pp. 405–23. Raven Press, New York.

Porter, R. W., Hohmann, G. W., Bors, E., and French, J. D. (1966). Cordotomy for pain following cauda equina injury. *Archives of Surgery*, **92**, 765–70.

Richardson, R. R., Meyer, P. R., and Cerullo, L. J. (1980). Neurostimulation in the modulation of intractable paraplegic and traumatic neuroma pains. *Pain*, **8**, 75–84.

Richter, H. P. and Seitz, K. (1984). Dorsal root entry zone lesions for the control of deafferentation pain: experiences in ten patients. *Neurosurgery*, **15**, 956–9.

Rose, M., Robinson, J. E., Ells, P., and Cole, J. D. (1988). Pain following spinal cord injury: results from a postal survey. *Pain*, **34**, 101–2.

Sindou, M. and Daher, A. (1988). Spinal cord ablation procedures for pain. In *Pain research and clinical management*, Vol. 3 (ed. R. Dubner, G. F. Gebhart, and M. R. Bond), pp. 477–95. Elsevier, Amsterdam.

Sindou, M., Fischer, G., Goutelle, A., and Mausuy, L. (1974). La radicellotomie posterieure selective. Premiers résultats dans la chirurgie de la douleur. *Neurochirurgie*, **20**, 391–408.

Tunks, E. (1986). Pain in spinal cord injured patients. In *Management of spinal cord injuries* (ed. R. F. Block and M. Basbaum), pp. 180–211. Williams & Wilkins, Baltimore.

Wall, P. D. (1978). The gate control theory of pain mechanisms. *Brain*, **101**, 1–18.

White, J. C. and Sweet, W. H. (1969). *Pain and the neurosurgeon*, pp. 633–887. Charles C. Thomas, Springfield, Illinois.

Wycis, H. T. and Spiegel, E. A. (1962). Long-range results in the treatment of intractable pain by stereotaxic midbrain surgery. *Journal of Neurosurgery*, **19**, 101–7.

Sexual function following spinal cord injury

B. P. Gardner and P. Rainsbury

Introduction

Spinal cord dysfunction is not limited to motor sensory and bladder problems, but includes the important aspect of sexuality. This may be ignored by the medical profession, but is never ignored by the patient. The patient with a spinal lesion may suffer a reduction in sexual attractiveness (real or imagined), with a concomitant psychological component of reduction in sexual drive or libido compounded by fear of rejection, pain, depression, and the possible effect of medication. Physical problems include difficulty or impossibility of movement, and the control of bodily functions, including sphincter control and stoma incontinence. The neurophysiological basis of sexual competence may be affected. Arousal, erection, ejaculation, and orgasm may be affected by neurological damage, aggravated by psychogenic and behavioural impotence. The circumstances of lack of mobility and privacy imposed upon a patient with spinal dysfunction will further limit sexual opportunities and encounters with the opposite sex. Many of these aspects can be ameliorated by early and continued counselling. Stimulation procedures may be necessary to achieve erection and ejaculation. These procedures are dealt with in the following chapter, but will also be discussed in more detail in a further volume on spinal dysfunction.

Fertility is a problem for both sexes, but in women fertility and the ability to have children is often relatively unaffected.

Sexual counselling

Counselling in all areas, but particular in sexual aspects, is vital. This should be made available at various times in the rehabilitation process as difficulties present. This will help to minimize sexual fears and personal doubts, as well as to enable the modern advances to be made available as appropriate. (Cole *et al.* 1973; Comarr and Vigue 1978.)

The first weekend home and the weeks following initial discharge are important sexual milestones. Appropriate guidance must be given in advance of these stages.

Following hospital discharge, a relationship comes under particular stress especially if the able-bodied partner is forced to take on the role of nurse and carer rather than that of spouse or lover. Continued support and regular follow-up of relationships, including sexual aspects, will help to minimize the stresses.

Different cultures and systems present different problems. The relevant approach will vary with the country and group concerned. Personal and moral issues require careful consideration.

Many spinal cord injured persons will not marry, but all need personal relationships. Sexual activity persists in spite of alteration in sexual responses, and is enjoyed by the majority of spinal cord injured patients (Guttmann 1964; Higgins 1979; Lowe and Carroll 185.)

Female spinal cord injured

Libido

In women this is related to psychodynamic factors in addition to physical ones. It may be reduced, but the emotional drive is unchanged.

Sexual intercourse

Tumescence of the clitoris and labia minora equates to erection, contraction of smooth muscle and the paraurethral glands of Skene to emission, and striated muscle contraction to ejaculation.

Taking the phases of Masters and Johnson (1965) and applying these to spinal cord injured women:

The resting phase

Women with complete lesions above T10 have total loss of internal organ and external genitalia sensitivity. Those from T12–S2 have partial insensitivity of internal organs, with total loss of sensation from external genitalia. Those from S2 to S5 have internal organ sensation and partial retention of external genitalia sensitivity.

Women with incomplete lesions retain varying degrees of sensation, with partial retention of pelvic-floor muscle control.

Excitation phase

This phase consists of lubrication, clitoral swelling, and labia congestion.

Women with lesions at T9 and above have reflex lubrication, reflex congestion with tactile stimuli (analogous to reflex erection), and some sensation in the excitation phase (burning in the urethra or fullness of the bladder).

Those between T10 and T12 have no lubrication, either reflex or psychogenic. No sensation is felt during this phase. Sympathetic nervous function is affected.

Those below T12 have psychogenic lubrication. Excitation phase is diminished.

Plateau phase

The clitoris retracts, with heightened tension in the genital area.

Women with complete lesions above T6 may experience autonomic hyperreflexia in this phase. Those complete above T10 occasionally have clitoral retraction with masturbation. Those between T10 and T12 have no sensation in this phase. Those below T12 have greatly attenuated sensation.

Orgasm

Women complete at T6 and above may experience autonomic dysreflexia. Those from between T10 and T12 have no sensation. Those below T12 have a deadened sensation that causes frustration.

Relaxation phase

Psychological activity accompanies sexual reactions. Fantasies can be created by spinal-cord-damaged women, and may be a very important part of sexual activity.

Problems associated with sexual intercourse

A. Spasticity may prevent penetration.

B. Deficient lubrication may prevent penetration. If reflex lubrication is triggered or lubricants are used this can be overcome.

Faecal or bladder incontinence may occur, either reflexly or following increased pressure. Voiding and evacuation prior to intercourse are recommended to avoid this. Indwelling catheters need not be removed, but they should be lubricated to avoid friction.

The incidence of urinary tract infection is increased by intercourse.

Fertility

Amenorrhoea is common following spinal cord injury. It usually lasts from three to nine months. Since the cycle phase is anovulatory in amenorrhoea, ovulation precedes the first period after injury. Since this may coincide with going home, great care must be taken if an unwanted pregnancy is to be avoided.

Following this initial stage normal reproductive capability is restored.

Pregnancy

This lasts the normal span. Close liaison between the spinal injuries specialist team and an obstetrics team experienced in the delivery of spinal-cord-damaged women is essential.

The pregnancy has several risks. Urinary tract infections may occur. A high fluid intake is recommended. Constipation, deep venous thrombosis, and increased osteoporosis are more common. Autonomic dysreflexia may arise in women with lesions above T7. Lower limb oedema may require support stockings. Premature labour may go unnoticed, and breaking of the waters may be confused with incontinence.

Uterine innervation is from T10 to T12 inclusive. Women with lesions above T10 feel no uterine contractions or fetal movements. Those whose lesions are T6 and above may experience fetal movements and uterine contractions as varying degrees of autonomic hyperreflexia. Those with lesions below T12 feel both uterine contractions and fetal movements.

Frequent examinations are required from 32 weeks onward, with admission to the spinal unit from week 36. (Axel 1982; Greenspoon and Paul 1986; Rossier *et al* 1969; Verduyn 1986.)

Delivery

This is best carried out in the obstetrics unit, with spinal specialist expertise being available to advise and anaesthetic support at hand to provide an epidural for those with lesions at T6 and above, to reduce the risk of autonomic hyperreflexia. Natural childbirth is the goal. Uterine contractions occur with lesions above T11. Those at T11 and T12 also have contractions, despite lacking reflex function, and deliver naturally. Those below T12 have uterine but no perineal sensation, so the risk of a vaginal tear is increased. (Young *et al.* 1983.)

Post partum

The mother should return to the spinal unit with her baby and remain until able to look after herself and her child without significant risk of developing a paraplegia-related complication. There is no contraindication to breast-feeding. Urinary tract infections and deep venous thrombosis may occur.

Motherhood

Many spinal-cord-injured women have successfully brought up children. In the early years, especially when the child is aged one to four years, particular problems exist, since the toddler is mobile but lacks the ability to reason, and therefore needs careful supervision which the paralysed mother canno readily provide. Extra care support should be provided at this time. (Turk *et al.* 1983.)

Male spinal cord injured

Libido

This remains strong in spinal-cord-injured men.

Erections

True erection comprises tumescence of the corpora cavernosa and corpus spongiosum. Priapism is tumescence of the corpora cavernosa only, not of the spongiosum of the urethra and glands. Vasodilatation of the arteries produces erection and retention of blood in the cavernous tissue by venous occlusion sustains it. Active venoconstriction may contribute in addition to passive compression of the subalbugineal venous plexus. Detumescence results from arterial vasoconstriction.

Psychogenic erections originate in visual, auditory, and olfactory sensation, recall, and perception. These act on the spinal cord via the brain. The efferent pathways are from the thoraco-lumbar and sacral erection centres.

Reflexogenic erections are elicited by exteroceptive (especially touching the skin of genitalia) and enteroceptive (for example, bladder) stimuli. The pelvic parasympathetic is involved in neural transmission, but the final common pathway is via short adrenergic nerves. (Lue and Tanagho 1987.)

Erections and neurological level

Patients with complete upper neuron lesions in respect of the sacral segments have exclusively reflexogenic erections, and occasionally no erections.

Those with incomplete upper motor neuron lesions may have reflexogenic and psychogenic erections.

Complete sacral lower motor neuron lesions may have psychogenic erections, but frequently have no erections.

Aids to erection/intercourse

While up to 70 per cent of spinal cord injured men may obtain erections, these are frequently irregular, ill-sustained, and insufficient for intercourse. Various adjunctive aids are available. Although penetration becomes possible with these, normal intercourse with orgasm will never be restored in patients with complete, and only in altered form in those with incomplete lesions. This must be carefully explained in the counselling that must precede the provision of these aids.

External aids. These devices, such as the erecaid and correctaid, depend on passive expansion of the penis either by an external cuff or by a vacuum, with the subsequent erection being maintained by a band around the base of the penis. These approaches are simple and non-invasive, and satisfy some couples. The risk that compression by the band may cause penile pressure sores must be explained.

Intracavernosal injections. Vasoactive drugs that cause arteriolar vasodilatation, including smooth-muscle relaxants such as papaverine and alpha-blocking agents such as phenoxybenzamine and phentolamine, will, if injected singly or in combination into the corpora cavernosa, cause these to engorge. The subsequent erection is abnormal in that the corpus spongiosum remains flaccid.

Using 1–2 ml syringes and with injections at various sites, 'erections' of different durations can be elicited. The appropriate dose will vary with the individual, but in all cases initial injections must be with small quantities of vasoactive drug.

Complications are few and rarely significant. These include ecchymoses, priapism (defined as erections lasting longer than 6 hours, and usually resolved by intracavernosal injection of phenylephrine or metaraminol), and fibrous nodules. Infection is very rare. (Bodner *et al.* 1987; Brindley 1983*a*; Brindley 1986; Hu *et al.* 1987; Wyndaele *et al.* 1986.)

Implants. A variety exist, including semi-rigid and inflatable types. These have not received widespread acceptance among patients or physicians. Complications occur, such as infection and erosion. With psychosexual counselling other methods of sexual expression may be found more appropriate than penile penetration, especially since this will never re-establish normal intercourse. (Green and Sloan 1986; Rossier and Fam 1984; Scott *et al.* 1973; Small *et al.* 1975.)

Sacral anterior root stimulator. In a significant proportion of patients, implant-driven erections may occur, in particular with S2 but also S2 root-stimulation. They have the advantages over intracavernosal injections of including corpus spongiosal in addition to corpus cavernosal tumescence, with consequently a more normal erection, and of the duration of each erection's being more readily controlled. The strengths of these erections may diminish with time.

Ejaculation

Ejaculation is the clonic contraction of the bulbo- and ischiocavernosus muscles, with associated movement of striated muscle of the pelvic floor, lower extremities, and trunk. Parasympathetic sacral outflow and somatic efferents account for this activity.

In the ejaculation reflex, afferent stimuli travel in the pudendal nerve (S2–S4) from the glans penis. Efferent stimuli travel along T11–L2 sympathetic preganglionic fibres via the hypogastric plexus and terminate on short postganglionic fibres in the prostate, seminal vesicles, and vas deferens. This sympathetic activity gives rise to contraction of these organs, and therefore emission. It also contracts the bladder-neck.

Ejaculation occurs rarely with upper motor neuron patients, occasionally being associated with reflex erections. It is more frequent with lower motor neuron lesions in association with psychogenic erections.

Incomplete spinal cord damaged patients ejaculate more frequently, usually in association wih reflex erections in upper motor neuron cases, and always with psychogenic erections in lower motor neuron cases.

Seminal emission

This comprises peristalsis of the smooth muscle of the vasa deferentia, prostate, seminal vesicles, and bladder-neck. It is mediated by the T11–L2 sympathetic nervous system.

Orgasm

Orgasm is a sensation that precedes and coincides with emission and ejaculation. It is rare with upper motor neuron lesions, though spasms may indicate that ejaculation has occurred. It is frequent with lower motor neuron patients, though sensation is referred to the groin, inner thigh, or lower abdomen, not the penis or urethra.

Methods for obtaining semen in spinal-cord-injured men

Electroejaculation

This induces semen emission, rarely ejaculation. It has been used in animals since the 1930s and in man since 1948. Myelinated preganglionic efferent sympathetic fibres from T11 to L2 inclusive are stimulated transrectally.

Using this method of transrectal electrostimulated semen emission Brindley has obtained semen from 97 out of 154 spinally injured men. Seven of the remainder might have provided semen under general anaesthesia, since pain prevented use of the device. A similar success-rate was obtained by Seager, most notably in thoracic spinal cord injured patients. (Kremer 1965, Halstead *et al.* Martin *et al.* 1983; Seager *et al.* 1984.)

Home electroejaculation by wives or the paraplegic man can be taught, but in general this is impractical.

Hypogastric stimulation

At laparotomy, the hypogastric plexus is isolated where it crosses the bifurcation of the aorta. It is then encircled by a cuff, which can subsequently be stimulated by a remote electrical device applied to the abdominal wall.

Erection and seminal emission occur following stimulation of the T11 to L2 sympathetic outflow.

Vibration

This was first applied to man by Comarr in 1970.

The optimum method uses the Ling vibrator at 80 Hz and with a peak-to-peak amplitude of 2.5 mm when loaded with the penis. The frenum is the most sensitive area.

Afferent fibres travel along the pudendal nerve (S2–S4). Central fibres then pass to the T11–L2 level to stimulate the preganglionic sympathetic fibres involved in emission and bladder-neck closure, and to parasympathetic and somatic efferents involved in ischiocavernosus, bulbocavernosus, and pelvic-floor muscle contractions.

Vibration rarely succeeds in the first six months following injury. It always fails in sole-scratch-negative patients. Sole-scratch-positive patients are those who have hip flexion (L2) in response to sole-scratch (S1).

Brindley obtained semen using the vibrator in 75 per cent of sole-scratch-positive patients over six months after injury. Significant autonomic hyperreflexia occurred in 7 of the 93 men, all except one (T2) being cervicals. Vibrator-failure men may produce semen with electrorectal stimulation. (Brindley 1981*a*, 184..)

The Ling vibrator may work where the Pifco (100 Hz and 1.2 mm amplitude) does not. Home vibration is practicable, provided that autonomic hyperreflexia does not occur, though this can still arise unexpectedly in men with lesions above T7 who have previously used this technique with no ill effect.

Using the vibrator and rectal electrostimulation, Brindley achieved 11 pregnancies (in 8 couples) after insemination of 21 wives. Semen was obtained by vibrator or electroejaculation in 51 per cent of his men. Later series report success-rates for obtaining semen of up to 91 per cent using his methods and equipment.

Semen capsule

This applies in those with no T11–L2 sympathetic efferent fibres in whom the vibrator and rectal electrostimulators will not be efficacious. It is also indicated where unacceptable levels of autonomic hyperreflexia occur with other approaches.

Permanent reservoirs are implanted into the subcutaneous tissues of the inguinal region. The vas deferentia are cannulated. Sperm can then be aspirated from these reservoirs, which are filled directly from the cannulated vasa. The couples are taught to aspirate the reservoirs themselves. (Brindley *et al.* 1986.)

Epididymal aspiration

This surgical technique involves extruding the scrotal contents through a small incision. The tunica vaginalis is opened, and the epididymis is exposed. Using an operating microscope, a tiny incision is made with the microscissors into the epididymal tunic to expose the tubules in the most distal portion of the epididymis. Sperm is aspirated with a syringe directly from the opening of the epididymal tubule. The fluid thus obtained is diluted with buffered media, and a portion is examined for motility and progression. If these parameters are poor, a further aspiration is made more proximally, and so on, until a sample with good progression and motility is obtained. This technique was originally applied to men with failed reversal of sterilization. Its place in spinal cord injured men is untested.

It has long been assumed that sperm must pass through a certain length of epididymis to mature, gain progressive motility, and become capable of fertilization. Other observations suggest that sperm may only require a period of time to mature after leaving the testicle.

Intrathecal neostigmine

An ejaculate may result, but as autonomic hyperreflexia may occur in men with lesions above T7 and may be difficult to control, this method is rarely used. (Spira 1958.)

Subcutaneous physostigmine

This method has been successful in producing an ejaculate. It can be applied by the couple at home. Side-effects are fewer than with intrathecal neostigmine, but the method is infrequently used as precise control is lacking. (Chapelle *et al.* 1983.)

Bladder-outlet surgery and fertility

Bladder-neck resection is associated with retrograde ejaculation. External sphincterotomy has no adverse effect on fertility.

Semen quality in spinal-cord-injured men

Three-quarters of normal men have 50 million motile sperm per ejaculate. The total normally motile normal-form sperm-count per ejaculate in spinal cord injured men is usually much less than this.

No close correlation between time since injury and the quality of semen after the first eight weeks have been demonstrated.

Retrograde ejaculates have fewer motile sperm than antegrade ejaculates, as urine is harmful to sperm. The quality of semen tends to improve with successive ejaculations following spinal injury, often over several months. Semen obtained using the vibrator is of better quality than that using rectal electrostimulation methods. The semen quality of spinal-cord-damaged men is reduced by raised scrotal temperature, which is due partly to the wheelchair position and in part to loss of lumbar sympathetic nerve supply, chronic infection, and non-drainage. (Brindley 1982.)

Semen-quality impairment in spinal-cord injured men is not related to oligoasthenospermia alone. Teratospermia may result from prolonged, recurring urinary tract infections. This reduces the number of normal forms available for fertilization.

Testicular histology

Tubular atrophy, interstitial sclerosis, and reduced spermatogenesis are common, especially in higher lesions. (Leriche *et al.* 1977; Morley *et al.* 1979; Perkash *et al.* 1985.)

Hormone changes

Urinary 17-ketosteroids and oestrogens are frequently elevated. A minority of patients have raised FSH levels, or an exaggerated FSH response to LHRH, a sensitive test of tubular damage.

Semen storage

Sperm density and motility diminishes dramatically in the early weeks following spinal cord damage. Ideally, semen should be collected before this loss of quality occurs. For a variety of reasons this is rarely possible, not least because of the unstable clinical condition of the patient in the immediate post-injury phase. At a later stage storage is less attractive, as motility will be reduced still further by this action.

The Stoke Mandeville Hospital/Bourn Hall Clinic programme for biological fatherhood in spinal-cord-injured men

Achieving the highest success for biological fatherhood for the spinal-cord-damaged patient depends on drawing together the three major components of modern spinal injury fertility treatment, via semen collection, semen preparation, and assisted conception. It is predicted that 70 per cent of all couples receiving treatment according to the algorithm of Fig. 10.1 will achieve biological parenthood. Using this scheme men with total motile counts as low as 30 000, a figure less than 0.01 per cent of normal, have achieved biological fatherhood.

With further developments, including the use of microinjection and micromanipulation, even smaller sperm numbers will probably prove

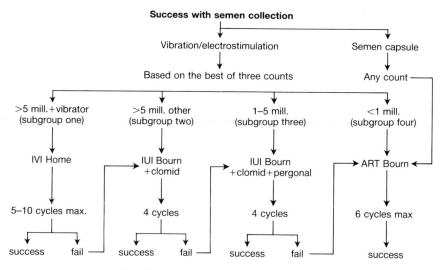

Fig. 10.1. Success with semen collection.

sufficient, raising the possibility of biological fatherhood for all spinal-cord-injured men with wives of child-bearing age.

The age of the woman is important. Younger women are more fertile. The risk of multiple pregnancy must be borne in mind, especially since caring for children is more difficult for the paralysed. The reduced life expectancy of the spinal-cord-damaged man increases the chance of any child's becoming prematurely fatherless. Full counselling is essential.

Semen collection

Couples are first assessed to determine the optimum method for semen collection. Then, according to this and the total normal-form normally motile count, they receive appropriate treatment so as to provide a good chance of biological parenthood within a reasonable number of cycles for any given couple.

Autonomic hyperreflexic treatment facilities must be available for couples above T7.

The optimum method for semen collection is the vibrator. Home vibration following advice on determining the fertile part of the cycle can be employed.

Rectal electrostimulation can be applied at home, but, because the techniques are more difficult and the Seager equipment so expensive, in practice it must be applied in the fertility centre.

The semen capsule is reserved for those from whom semen cannot be obtained by vibration or electroejaculation. Because the capsule may have spermicidal qualities, and the risk of infection is ever-present, such couples should immediately enter the assisted reproduction technique (ART) group.

The hypogastric stimulator, with or without the sacral anterior root stimulator, is not a part of the programme at present, given its invasive character and the relatively high success of other methods for semen collection.

Epididymal aspiration has not yet been well developed in the United Kingdom, but remains a possibility for those in whom the semen capsule is unsuccessful.

Semen preparation

Following ovulation-induction for artificial insemination, or successful collection of oocytes for *in vitro* fertilization (IVF) or gamete intra-Fallopian transfer (GIFT), the semen must be prepared for insemination. The aim of semen preparation is to separate sperm from seminal plasma. This contains inhibitors which prevent capacitation. It also contains agents which, if introduced into the uterus, may cause a severe inflammatory response.

By a process of layering using culture medium, a population of motile sperm is obtained which is free from unwanted constituents of the raw ejaculate, such as non-motile sperm, cells, seminal plasma, and coagulum. The motile sperm are centrifuged to form a pellet, which can be re-suspended and washed several times.

Sperm agglutination is generally caused by the presence of sperm antibodies. These may be present in spinal-cord-damaged men. This problem may be overcome by the use of a medium containing a high concentration of serum protein obtained from the wife's serum prior to oocyte recovery. This coats the sperm surface and prevents agglutination.

Excessively viscous specimens are collected into culture medium. In such cases, the preparation is first centrifuged, and the supernatant is removed. Medium is placed on top of the sperm pellet. This is left for an hour, during which time motile sperm swim out of the pellet and into the medium.

Other methods may be used to improve sperm concentration in oligo-asthenospermia. These include specialized centrifugation of the semen sample, using more force, but in two concentrations of a buoyant medium which both prevents physical damage to the sperm and separates out motile sperm from the rest, probably because they adopt a steamlined alignment in the centrifugal field.

The aim with IVF is to produce a stock of 500 000 motile sperm per ml. This is diluted for insemination of the oocyte to around 100 000 motile sperm per millilitre. Each oocyte is placed in a drop of 0.25 ml of this preparation for fertilization to occur. (Steptoe and Edwards 1978.)

Female treatment

Artificial insemination. Assuming that a reasonable sperm preparation can be obtained by the methods described, the first step towards assisted reproduction in these couples is artificial insemination. In its simplest form this involves identifying the time of ovulation by serial ultrasound examinations in a normal cycle, followed by intravaginal or intrauterine insemination. Intravaginal insemination can be easily carried out in a home setting. Intrauterine insemination requires sperm-washing, in order to remove seminal plasma.

Artificial insemination procedures are only one-fifth as effective in generating a pregnancy per cycle treatment as the 'high-tech' methods of *in vitro* fertilization and gamete intra-Fallopian transfer described below.

Normal human fertility depends upon the successful fertilization of an oocyte at the distal end of the Fallopian tube, and its subsequent transport to the uterus, culminating in implantation.

The original indication for attempting *in vitro* fertilization (IVF) was to bypass blocked Fallopian tubes. Louise Brown's birth in 1978 followed the successful fertilization of a single oocyte collected from one ovarian follicle in a natural cycle.

Recent advances in ovarian stimulation protocols now produce multiple follicular development yielding several oocytes rather than one. This allows more than one embryo to be replaced at embryo transfer (ET), thus increasing the chance of successful implantation.

In vitro *fertilization (IVF) and gamete intra-Fallopian transfer (GIFT).* These two techniques together represent the 'high-tech' assisted reproduction procedures available today. Both involve the same ovarian stimulation protocols in the female, culminating in oocyte retrieval, generally by the vaginal ultrasound-directed route in IVF, or by laparoscopy in GIFT.

Follicular development is achieved in both techniques using similar protocols; 95 per cent of patients today are treated with the luteinizing-hormone-releasing-hormone agonist (the GnRH analogue) in conjunction with gonadotrophins. This GnRH analogue [SUPREFACT 'Buserelin'] produces pituitary 'down-regulation' and de-sensitization. (Howles *et al.* 1987.)

Oocyte recovery and IVF/GIFT results. Oocyte recovery in IVF is accomplished using ultrasound-guided techniques, most commonly by the vaginal route. Oocytes are retrieved using a fine aspirating needle connected to a vacuum system. The oocytes are harvested 35 hours following human chorionic gonadotrophin administration [Profasi 5000 IU] with the patient under light anaesthesia, and usually between days 10 and 12 of the artificial cycle. An average of 7 oocytes per patient is collected.

Provided oocyte and sperm quality are good, 80 per cent fertilization-rates can be achieved. Forty-eight hours later 3–4 embryos are replaced (without anaesthesia) into the uterine cavity via a transfer catheter to a depth of 5 cm from the external cervical os.

Pregnancy rates of 25 per cent or better per transfer are now achieved in most units, with a 'Take-home baby' rate of 20 per cent for IVF, after allowing for spontaneous abortion, ectopic pregnancy, and late pregnancy complications.

Gamete intra-Fallopian transfer (GIFT). This procedure can be regarded as '*in vivo* fertilization', as opposed to '*in vitro* fertilization'. The woman must have at least one patent, healthy Fallopian tube. Following ovarian follicular stimulation and appropriately-timed HCG administration, oocytes are collected laparoscopically. The embryologist selects the best 3 or 4 oocytes, and these, together with a preparation of the husband's semen, are placed directly into the distal ends of one or both Fallopian tubes to a depth of 2 cm, using a transfer catheter inserted through the abdominal wall under laparoscopic vision. This optimizes the chance of oocytes and sperm fertilizing in the natural situation and at the correct time of the cycle.

The pregnancy rate following the GIFT procedure can be as high as 40 per cent in carefully selected cases, especially in unexplained infertility.

If more than four oocytes are collected (referred to as 'spare eggs'), the surplus are put for *in vitro* fertilization. Should these spare eggs successfully fertilize, then the healthy embryos generated are frozen for subsequent replacement in a natural cycle. If the GIFT procedure is not successful, or if the couple wish for a further pregnancy, the frozen embryos can be thawed and replaced at a later date.

Ovarian follicular stimulation protocols in IVF and GIFT. Two regimes in common use are:

1. *The long buserelin–gonadotrophin regime (LBG)*. Buserelin is administered in a dose of 500 micrograms subcutaneously daily from the luteal phase of the previous menstrual cycle prior to the IVF treatment cycle (i.e.: day 23 of a 28-day cycle). A baseline ultrasound pelvic scan and biochemical profile, consisting of serum oestradiol, luteinizing hormone, and progesterone levels is carried out on day 2 of the IVF cycle. If these parameters indicate that successful 'down-regulation' of the pituitary has been achieved then daily intramuscular injections of purified human menopausal gonadotrophin [HMG—'Pergonal' (Serono)] are administered to promote follicular growth and maturation. However, is most cases ovulation and luteinization will not occur without an additional injection of HCG [human chorionic gonadotrophin—'Profasi' (Serono)]. This stimulates the LH surge, and thus produces luteinization and ripening of the oocytes. Oocyte retrieval is carried out around day 12 of the cycle.

2. *The short buserelin–gonadotrophin regime (SBG)*. The rationale of this regime, which is currently providing the best pregnancy rates at Bourn Hall, is to provoke enhanced gonadotrophin secretion by direct pituitary gland stimulation by the LHRH agonist.

This produces follicular recruitment during the critical period in the early stages of the menstrual cycle, but does not sustain the hypersecretion into the critical stages of pre-ovulatory development. Although there do not appear to be any microscopic differences in oocyte quality, the suppression of LH levels in plasma in the late follicular phase of SBG-treated patients suggests that the degree of exposure of the follicle to LH is reduced. The resulting oocytes collected are of optimal maturity, and produce fitter embryos which have a greater chance of implanting.

Oocyte micromanipulation techniques. In severe oligoasthenospermia, where counts are consistently lower than 300 000 per ml and motility less than 15 per cent, mechanical disruption (drilling or cutting), or enzymatic dissolution of the zona pellucida (zona stripping) may enhance fertilizing capacity. (Edwards and Rainsbury 1988.)

Microinjection, which is the injection of one or more individual sperms directly into the peri-vitelline space of the oocyte, may overcome the problem of severe oligospermia.

References

Amelar, R. D., *et al.* (1982). Sexual function and fertility in paraplegic males. *Urology*, **20**(1), 62–5.

Axel, S. (1982). Spinal cord injured women's concerns: menstruation and pregnancy. *Nursing*, **10**, 10–15.

Bennett, C. J., Seager, S. W., Vasher, E. A., and McGuire, E. J. (1988). Sexual dysfunction and ejaculation in men with spinal cord injury: review. *Journal of Urology*, **139**, 453–7.

Berard, D. J. J. (1989). The sexuality of spinal cord injured women: physiology and pathophysiology. A review. *Paraplegia*, **27**, 99–112.

Bodner, D. R., Lindan, R., Leffler, E., Kursh, E. D., and Resnick, M. I. (1987). The application of intracavernosal injection of vasoactive medications for erection in men with spinal cord injury. *Journal of Urology*, **138**, 310–11.

Bors, E. and Comarr, A. E. (1960). Neurological disturbance of sexual function with special reference to 529 patients with spinal cord injury. *Urological Survey*, **10**, 191–222.

Brindley, G. S. (1981*a*). Reflex ejaculation under vibratory stimulation in paraplegic men. *Paraplegia*, **19**(5), 299–302.

Brindley, G. S. (1981*b*). Electroejaculation: its technique, neurological implications and uses. *Journal of Neurology, Neurosurgery, and Psychiatry*, **44**, 9–18.

Brindley, G. S. (1982). Deep scrotal temperature and the effect on it of clothing, air temperature, activity, posture and paraplegia. *British Journal of Urology*, **54**, 49–55.

Brindley, G. S. (1983*a*). Cavernosal alpha blockade: a new technique for investigating and treating erectile impotence. *British Journal of Psychiatry*, **143**, 332–7.

Brindley, G. S. (1983*b*). Physiology of erection and management of paraplegic infertility. In *Male infertility* (ed. T. B. Hargreave), pp. 261–79. Springer Verlag, Berlin.

Brindley G. S., (1984). The fertility of men with spinal injuries. *Paraplegia*, **22**, 337–48.

Brindley, G. S. (1986). Maintenance treatment of erectile impotence by cavernosal unstriated muscle relaxant injection. *British Journal of Psychiatry*, **149**, 210–15.

Brindley, G. S., Scott, G. I., and Hendry, W. F. (1986). Vas cannulation with implanted sperm reservoirs for obstructive azoospermia or ejaculatory failure. *British Journal of Urology*, **58**, 721–3.

Chapelle, P. A., Blanquart, F., Puech, A. J., and Held, J. P. (1983). Treatment of anejaculation in the total paraplegic by subcutaneous injection of physostigmine. *Paraplegia*, **21**, 30.

Cole. T. M., Chilgren, R., and Rosenberg, P. (1973). A new programme of sex education and counselling for spinal cord injured adults and health care professionals. *Paraplegia*, **11**, 111.

Comarr, A. E. (1971). Sexual concepts in traumatic cord and cauda equina lesions. *Journal of Urology*, **106**, 375.

Comarr, A. E. (1985). Sexuality and fertility among spinal cord and/or cauda equina injuries. *Journal of the American Paraplegia Society*, **8**, 67–75.

Comarr, E. and Vigue, M. (1978). Sexual counselling among male and female patients with spinal cord and/or cauda equina injury. *American Journal of Physical Medicine*, **57**, 107.

Crich, J. P. and Jequier, A. M. (1978). Infertility in men with retrograde ejaculation: the action of urine on sperm motility, and a simple method for achieving antegrade ejaculation. *Fertility and Sterility*, **30**, 572–6.

Edwards, R. G. and Rainsbury, P. A. (1988). Unpublished data—results of a 1988 micromanipulation trial at Bourn Hall.

Eliasson, R. (1971). Standards for investigation of human semen. *Andrologie*, **3**, 49–64.

François, N. and Maury, M. (1987). Sexual aspects in paraplegic patients. *Paraplegia*, **25**, 289–92.

Frankel, H. L., Mathias, C. J., and Walsh, J. J. (1979). Blood pressure, plasma catecholamines and prostaglandins during artificial erection in a male tetraplegic. *Paraplegia*, **12**, 205.

Freud, M. (1962). Interrelationships among characteristics of human semen and factors effecting semen—specimen quality. *Journal of Reproduction and Fertility*, **4**, 143–7.

Friedman-Becker, E. (1977). *Female sexuality following paraplegia*. Cheever Publishing Edit, Bloomington, Illinois.

Gardner, B. P., Rainsbury, P. A., and Moffatt, B. (1990). *Collaborative trial between Stoke Mandeville Spinal Injuries Unit and Bourn Hall IVF clinic*.

Gillan, P. and Brindley, G. S. (1979). Vaginal and pelvic floor responses to sexual stimulation. *Psychophysiology*, **16**, 471–81.

Green, B. G. and Sloan, S. L. (1986). Penile prosthesis in spinal cord injured patients: combined psychosexual counselling and surgical regimen. *Paraplegia*, **24**, 167–72.

Greenspoon, J. S. and Paul, R. H. (1986). Paraplegia and quadriplegia: special considerations during pregnancy and labor and delivery. *American Journal of Obstetrics and Gynaecology*, **155**, 738–41.

Guttmann, L. (1949). The effect of prostigmine on the reproductive functions in spinal man. *Proceedings of the 4th International Neurological Congress, Vol. 2*, p. 69. Masson, Paris.

Guttmann, L. (1964). The married life of paraplegics and tetraplegics. *Paraplegia*, **2**, 182.

Guttmann, L. and Walsh, J. J. (1971). Prostigmine assessment test of fertility in spinal man. *Paraplegia*, **1**, 39–50.

Halstead, L. S., VerVoort, S., and Seager, S. W. J. (1987). Rectal probe electrostimulation in the treatment of anejaculatory spinal cord injured men. *Paraplegia*, **25**, 120.

Higgins, G. E. (jun.) (1979). Sexual response in spinal cord injured adults: a review of the literature. *Archives of Sexual Behavior*, **8**, 173.

Horne, H. W., Paull, D. P., and Munro, D. (1948). Fertility studies in human male with traumatic injuries of the spinal cord and cauda equina. *New England Journal of Medicine*, **239**, 959–61.

Howles, C. M., Macnamee, M. C., and Edwards, R. G. (1987). Pregnancies after IVF when high tonic LH is reduced by long-term treatment with GnRH agonists. *Human Reproduction*, **2**, 569.

Hu, K. N., Burks, C., and Christy, W. C. (1987). Fibrosis of tunica albuginea: complication of long-term intracavernous pharmacological self-injection. *Journal of Urology*, **138**, 404–5.

Kremer, J. (1965). A simple sperm penetration test. *International Journal of Fertility*, **10**, 209–15.

Leriche, A., Berard, E., Vauzelle, J. L., Minaire, P., Girard, R., Archimbaud, J. P., and Bourret, J. (1977). Histological and hormonal testicular changes in spinal cord injured patients. *Paraplegia*, **15**, 274–9.

Lowe, J. and Carroll, D. (1985). The effects of spinal cord injury on the intensity of emotional experience. *British Journal of Clinical Psychology*, **24**, 135–6.

Lue, T. F. and Tanagho, E. A. (1987). Physiology of erection and pharmacological management of impotence. *Journal of Urology*, **137**, 829–36.

Martin, E. E., Warner, H., Crenshaw, T. L., Crenshaw, R. T., Shapiro, C. E., and Perkash, I. (1983). Initiation of erection and semen release by rectal probe electrostimulation. *Journal of Urology*, **129**, 637–41.

Masters, W. H. and Johnson, V. E. (1965). *Human sexual response*, pp. 65–130. Little, Brown, and Co., Boston.

Morley, J. E., Distiller, L. A., Lissoos, I., Lipschitz, R., Kay, G., Searle, D. L. *et al.* (1979). Testicular function in patients with spinal cord damage. *Hormone and Metabolic Research*, **11**, 679.

Perkash, J., Martin, D. E., Warner, H., Blank, M. S., and Collins, D. C. (1985). Reproductive biology of paraplegics: results of semen collection, testicular biopsy and serum hormone evaluation. *Journal of Urology*, **134**, 284–8.

Rossier, A. B. and Fam, B. A. (1984). Indications and results of semi-rigid penile prostheses in spinal cord injury patients: longterm followup. *Journal of Urology*, **131**, 59–61.

Rossier, A. B., Ruffieux, M., and Ziegler, W. H. (1969). Pregnancy and labour in high traumatic spinal cord lesions. *Paraplegia*, **7**, 210–16.

Scott, F. B., Bradley, W. E., and Tim, G. W. (1973). Management of erectile impotence. Use of implantable, inflatable prostheses. *Urology*, **2**, 80–2.

Seager, S. W., Savastano, J. A., Streett, J. W., Halstead, L., and McGuire, E. J. (1974). Electroejaculation, semen quality, and penile erections in normal and chronic spinal non-human primates. *Journal of Urology*, **131**(2), 234a, abstract 522.

Silber, S. J. Pregnancy after vasovasostomy for vasectomy reversal: a study of factors affecting long-term return of fertility in 282 patients followed for ten years. *Human Reproduction*. (In press.)

Small, M. P., Carrion, H. M., and Gordon, J. A. (1975). Small–Carrion penile prosthesis. *Urology*, **5**, 479–86.

Spira, R. (1958). Artificial insemination after intrathecal injection of neostigmine in a paraplegic. *Lancet*, **i**, 670.

Steptoe, P. C. and Edwards, R. G. (1978). Birth after the reimplantation of a human embryo. *Lancet*, **ii**, 366.

Turk, R., Turk, M., and Assejev, V. (1983). The female paraplegic and mother–child relations. *Paraplegia*, **21**, 186–91.

Verduyn, W. H. (1986). Spinal cord injured women; pregnancy and delivery. *Paraplegia*, **24**, 231–40.

Weber, D. K. and Wessman, H. C. (1971). A review of sexual function following spinal cord trauma. *Physical Therapy*, **51**, 290.

Wyndaele, J. J., DeMeyer, J. M., De Sy, W. A., and Claessens, H. (1986). Intra-cavernous injection of vasoactive drugs, an alternative for treating impotence in spinal cord injury patients. *Paraplegia*, **24**, 271–5.

Young, B. K., Katz, M., and Klein, S. (1983). Pregnancy after spinal cord injury. Altered maternal and fetal responses to labor. *Obstetrics and Gynaecology*, **62**, 59–65.

Zeitlin, A. B., Cottrell, T. L., and Lloyd, F. A. (1957). Sexology of the paraplegic male. *Fertility and Sterility*, **8**, 337–44.

III

Behavioural therapy

11

Current ideas on motor control and learning: implications for therapy
Theo Mulder

How are movements controlled?

Each day we perform thousands of movements, almost without effort or attention. Everything looks so easy for the normal, healthy adult; but we have forgotten the trouble a young child has with 'simple' motor skills such as walking, eating, holding a glass, regulating balance, reaching, climbing, etc. We have forgotten the thousands of repetitions necessary for mastering these skills. However, when observing a patient suffering from the consequences of damage to the motor system, we immediately realize the vulnerability of the system and the fact that it is only 'one step' from the highly skilled smooth performance of the healthy adult to the impaired invalid motor behaviour of the patient.

Motor control is a complex process. consider, for example, the following simple skill, viz. the active catching of a ball. When analysing this task in terms of information processes it becomes clear that even such a simple task comprises a large number of processes.

Cognitive/motor processes which may play a role in the skill of catching a ball
— the instruction must be understood
— the instruction must be stored in memory for a short time (STM function)
— attention span must be sufficient
— visual fixation of the object
— identification of the object as a ball
— adequate perception of the trajectory of the ball
— co-ordination movement of head and eyes
— knowledge of body position (processing of proprioceptive and exproprioceptive information)
— selection of the adequate response
— linking of the actual response to similar responses performed in the past (LTM function)
— retrieval of a raw, prototypical action schema from long-term memory

— the adjustment of the raw action schema to the actual requirements (such as force, velocity, accuracy)
— regulation of balance
— the co-ordination of agonistic and antagonistic muscles
— start of the movement
— processing of feedback
— correction of the movement in progress on the basis of processed afferent feedback
— STOP
— processing of knowledge of results
— start of a new attempt

This example clearly shows that motor control is a multi-layered process. There are no ready-made efferent instructions regulating the movement in a strictly 'top-down' order, but the movement is *constructed* on the basis of several streams of input.

This example has implications for the diagnosis of motor disorders, since it indicates that observed problems in the overt motor output can be understood in terms of disorders of one (or more) of the above-mentioned processes (the application of such a process-oriented approach to the diagnosis of motor disorders has been described elsewhere—Hulstijn and Mulder 1985, 1986; Mulder *et al.* 1986.

One of the most interesting sources of input is the perceptual input.

Perception and action

Traditionally the visual system has been described as an exteroceptor (as a source of extrinsic information). It was thought of as a receptor that provides information only about the movements of other objects in the environment. Although it does have this capability, it has been indicated recently that the eye can also function as a proprioceptor. These recent notions are strongly influenced by the work of Gibson (1979), who considered vision as a far richer source of information than is implied by passive registration of events in the environment. Think of the retina as being bombarded with rays of light from the objects in the visual field. The locations that these rays find on the retina are unique for each position that an eye can achieve in space. Moving the head changes the angles of entry of these rays into the eye and hence relative locations on the retina. For example, as I sit here and I move my head slightly to the left I see the computer screen also move relative to a particular place on the wall behind the screen. If I move my head downward I perceive predictable changes in the visual scene again (see Schmidt 1988, p. 149).

The pattern of rays experienced in this way is termed the *optical array* and it provides a unique specification of the location of the eye in space. The

hanges in the optical array when the eye is moved from one place to another
re called the *optical flow*. The crucial point is that vision provides not only
n indication of movements in the outside world but is also a rich source of
nformation concerning our own movements in that world. The moving
ptical flow not only tells me about my movements in the environment, but it
lso tells me about the environment in ways that I could not achieve if I were
ot moving at all (see Schmidt 1988, p. 150).

Hence vision is not merely an exteroceptive sense, passively informing the
ubject about changes in the environment, but is also a proprioceptive sense
elling the subject about his own movements. Against this backgound Lee
1980) argued that we should add the term *exproprioception* to Sherrington's
riginal list (interoceptive, exteroceptive, proprioceptive).

In the Gibsonian (or ecological) view, movement and vision are very
losely and reciprocally linked. For example, it is stated that visual informa-
on plays an essential role in the regulation of movements, particularly in the
aintenance of balance.

Standing (but also sitting) involves continuous compensatory adjustments
f the musculature. Any sway of the body away from the vertical has to be
egistered, and compensatory muscular adjustments have to be made to
revent that balance's being lost. The classical view is that information about
osture comes from receptors in the vestibular canals and in the joints and
uscles particularly of the ankles and hips. According to this view, distur-
ances in balance are primarily compensated by means of reflex processes.
ven if the eye is involved at all in balance, it is of minor importance
ompared with the mechanoreceptors, since one can stand in the dark.
lowever, this classical view can be criticized, since there is growing experi-
ental evidence that vision does play a crucial role in the regulation of move-
ent. Lee and Aronson (1974) showed this in a beautiful experiment. They
sed the so-called *moving room*. The experimental situation was as follows.
ubjects (in these experiments children of the age of between 13 and 18
onths) were standing on a stationary floor with their face towards a wall,
ith a picture on it to make it more interesting. The experimental room,
omprising three walls and a ceiling, could be moved forward or backward
ast the subject standing on the stationary floor.

Consider a subject standing still in the room facing the closed end. Motion
f the room forward in the direction he is facing will produce optic flow
atterns that are similar to what would normally be perceived with backward
way. If he uses visual proprioception in maintaining posture, the visual
formation should induce muscular action to produce compensatory
rward torque. The converse holds for backward motion of the room. The
sults indicated that this was exactly what happened. A forward movement
f the room resulted in a forward sway or fall of the body, a backward
ovement, that is to say a movement towards the subject, resulted in falling

backwards. These results are interesting, since they indicated the dominan of visual information compared to the information coming from t mechanoreceptors. Remember that the floor was stationary, and hence changes occurred in proprioceptive information coming from the recepto in the ankle joints. Similar results were obtained with younger children wl were capable of sitting but not standing (Butterworth and Hicks 197' These experiments seem to indicate that, for infants at least, visual propri ceptive information is more potent than mechanical proprioceptive inform tion. In more recent experiments performed by Lee and his co-workers it h been found that adults show similar behaviour to that of infants. The effe was found even when the experimenter warned the subject that he was goi to try to make him sway by moving the room, and that he should do his best resist this by ignoring the room movement.

The role of visual information was further explored in a series of oth experiments. Lee *et al.* (1982) studied the behaviour of long-jumpers. In tl long-jump the athlete springs 30 to 40 m and has to leap off a narrow take-o board (20 cm wide). The accuracy of foot placement is essential. Tr athlete's toe needs to be as close as possible to the front edge of the boar since it is from this point that the length of the jump is measured. Hence, tr act of long-jumping is a very demanding task. It is therefore surprising ho accurately skilled long-jumpers can strike the take-off board. The standar error of the athletes in the study was about 8 cm.

How do they perform such a task, how do they adjust their strides to tr visually received take-off board, or in other words how do they determine tr time-to-contact with the board? What form of visual information do the use?

To answer this question the reader should recall the concepts of *optic array* and *optical flow*. Lee's very interesting statement is that the time-t contact (Tc) can be determined by changes in the optical flow. When tr dilation of the retinal image of the take-off board exceeds a critical value the certain motor systems are triggered. In another study Lee and Beddis investigated the behaviour of gannets diving into the sea. The birds div steeply from up to 100 ft with their wings partly open to steer themselves, an just before they reach the water surface (at up to 50 mph) they streamlin their bodies by stretching their wings right back and go in like a spear. Agai the question is how do they know when to streamline themselves for entry, o in other words, how is perception coupled to action? Also in this case it coul be indicated that the birds were using the same strategy as the long-jumper When the dilation of the water surface exceeded a critical value then the stetched their wings (Lee and Reddish 1981).

It is clear that a similar mechanism can be assumed for the human bein catching a ball, or steering a car or a wheelchair, or for a person regulating h or her balance. Changes in the optical flow inform the subject about move

ents of the body relative to the environment so that compensatory
easures can be taken.

From these and other behavioural experiments it is clear that vision can be
ewed as an integral component of the motor control system. Besides this
ere is also a growing body of physiological evidence for the existence of
st-acting visual–spinal pathways (see Nashner and Berthoz 1978). For
ample, it has been found that optical information specific to a cat's orienta-
on influences the activity in the cat's spinal motoneurons. A large disk of
loured dots was rotated in front of a cat's line of sight to imitate the optical
ow that would result from tilting. When the disk was rotated to the left
mulating a tilt to the right), the extensor reflexes on the right side of the cat
ere enhanced and the flexor reflexes on the left side were enhanced
hoden *et al.* 1977).

However, the data were not unequivocal. For example, Brandt *et al.*
976) did not succeed in producing an opto-kinetic effect in 6–12-year-old
ildren. Also the conclusion of Lee and Aronson (1974) and Kelso (1982)
at the infant's visual system is more highly developed and more reliable
an its proprioceptive system needs some reply. Woollacott (1986)
dicated that the proprioceptive activation of postural muscles seems to be
e-wired, and becomes functional prior to the visual system. She showed
at in four-months-old infants consistent and directionally appropriate neck
usculature became apparent when vision was *removed.* Also the Gibsonian
aim of perceptual dominance is not without problems. Dichgans *et al.*
974) and Young *et al.* (1975) indicated that the visually induced tilt
creased markedly when the otoliths are placed in a less favourable position
lateral head-tilt, indicating a more hybrid control system.

However, in spite of the sometimes contradictory results concerning the
ecise mechanisms it seems wise to emphasize the clinical importance of the
lationship between perception and action. It is clear that perceptional
sorders have an impact on motor control (see also Bles and Brandt 1986).
herefore the assessment of this relationship (also in terms of optic flow
tterns) deserves more attention in rehabilitation medicine. Several authors
dicated alterations of visual perception in a large number of patients with
ain damage (van Ravensberg *et al.* 1984) as well as disturbed balance
gulation (Hocherman and Dickstein 1984).

Besides this, it should be recognized that impairment of visual perception
rms an important limiting factor in the effectiveness of rehabilitation
incoln *et al.* 1985).

Up to now this assessment has received relatively little attention in the
rmal medical examination of patients suffering from the consequences of
mage to the central nervous system.

Motor learning

Rehabilitation can for a large part be conceived as a learning proce Learning refers to relatively stable changes in behaviour as a result practice. But *what* is learned when a patient becomes more skilful, has learned to control his *muscles* in a more efficient way, or has he learn particular *movements*, or has he learned *internal references* or *motor pr grammes*? In this section an attempt is made to answer this question. T answer has direct relevance for rehabilitation therapy, and indicates that many cases therapy takes place in a rather obsolete way.

Motor learning: the acquisition of internal references (the closed loop notion)

Adams (1971) presented a theory which he termed a *closed loop theory motor control.* This theory implies that the continuous availability of senso feedback is necessary for motor control. Any sizeable deficit in the flow organization of afferent information (both proprioceptive and exteroceptiv will result in a disturbance of skilled motor performance. In his terms, mot learning can be understood as the acquisition of a memory trace and perceptual trace for the movement under training. The memory trace can I understood as a 'mechanism', whose role it is to select and initiate tl response. The memory trace is, in fact, a motor programme operati without feedback (the term motor programme will be explained further in tl text). Its only function is to start the movement. The strength of the memo trace grows as a function of practice and feedback. The perceptual trace ca be viewed as a reference for adjustment of movements on the basis received peripheral feedback. This perceptual trace is fundamental f Adams's learning theory: it is the internal reference for the correct mov ment. During therapy this perceptual trace develops and becomes mo precise as a result of sensory feedback. Proprioception forms an essenti source of sensory feedback, but visual, auditory, and tactile information a also important for the development of the perceptual trace. The more fee back is available, the stronger becomes the perceptual trace, and the mo efficient the process of error detection. Especially during the first phase the therapy—or learning—process (which is called the verbal motor stag when the perceptual trace has to be developed, feedback is essential. Tl feedback is used to make the next response different from the previous or The mechanism responsible for evaluating the correctness of a particul response develops as a function of the sensory feedback impinging upon Without precise feedback the perceptual trace cannot be developed, forms only a 'weak' reference. Such a reference is a poor guide for respons and the result will be that performance hardly improves.

In Adams' framework therapy/training is the repetition of correct responses to strengthen the perceptual trace, whereby the therapist/training functions as the primary supplier of feedback.

Research indicated that when precision is required, as in relatively slow, goal-directed movements, such as reaching for a glass, the concept of a feedback system, comparing the output of the system with an internal reference value (the perceptual trace) is necessary, since corrections may be needed during the trajectory of the movement. However, it also indicated that with very fast, ballistic movements the notion of feedback as described above is limited in effectiveness.

Motor learning: the acquisition of motor programmes (the open loop notion)

Consider a very rapid movement, in which the pattern of action is initiated and completed in 100 to 200 msec. There are many examples of movements like this in sports—take for example the batswing in baseball (100 msec) or Muhammed Ali's left jab (40 msec). Feedback processes as suggested by Adams seem too sluggish for this type of control. Hence, in these cases it seems logical to assume that the central nervous system is capable of specifying the movement before it actually starts. The movement seems to be pre-programmed. A beautiful example of this can be found in an experiment performed by Wadman *et al.* (1979). Subjects had to perform rapid elbow extensions so that the hand came to rest in or near a target area. EMG's were recorded from the agonistic (m. triceps) and antagonistic (m. biceps) muscles. The results show the well-known three-burst pattern. This was the normal condition (see Fig. 11.1).

However, sometimes the movement was blocked (of course the subject did not know this beforehand). The subject attempted to start the movement, but this was impossible. Now, look at Fig. 11.1, there is something very interesting. When the curves 'normal' and 'blocked' are compared it can be observed that during the first 100 msec they do not differ. How can this be explained?

The best explanation is that (part of) the action pattern has been pre-programmed, structured in advance, and runs off as a unit without much possibility of modification from events in the environment. The results of Wadman *et al.* are a strong indication for the existence of a motor programme.

Traditionally the motor programme has been defined as a sequence of stored commands that 'is structured before the movement begins and allows the entire sequence to be carried out uninfluenced by peripheral feedback' (Keele 1968, p.387). However, although this might be the case in fast, highly overlearned movements, a strict application to all movements is

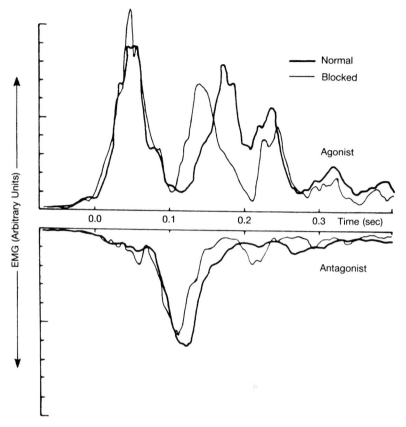

Fig. 11.1. shows the integrated EMG activity. The normal curve represents the condition in which the extension movement was possible. The blocked curve represents the condition in which the movement did not take place. Note that during the first 100 msec the curves are almost identical (from Wadman *et al.* 1979).

unacceptable, since for human beings there is no convincing evidence that *sequences* of movements can be performed without feedback. This does not imply that motor programmes do not exist, but it implies that the concept should be defined in a less strictly feedback-independent sense.

According to this notion learning is the acquisition of motor programmes. The problem for the subject in learning motor skills is to develop these open loop programmes to free one's self from feedback involvement. Pew (1966) has shown, in a task requiring alternate finger-tapping movements to keep a dot central on the screen, that there was a clear shift from closed-loop (feedback-dependent) to open-loop control.

Fundamental problems with closed-loop and open-loop theories

There are three fundamental and closely related problems (see also Mulder and Hulstijn 1984). First, I shall describe these problems and subsequently I will discuss a possible solution. The three problems are: *the problems of the degrees of freedom*; *the flexibility (or novelty) problem* and *the storage problem*.

The problem of the degrees of freedom

This problem was mentioned by Bernstein (1967). It is concerned with the very complex and unconstrained mechanical properties of the musculo-skeletal system: the number of different ways of moving—the degree of freedom—is huge for most movements. The higher levels of the central nervous system cannot be charged with specifying all the possible details, with the whole set of possible commands. The question now is: how can such a flexible system be controlled?

The flexibility (or novelty) problem

This problem refers to the fact that the same movement patterns can be performed with different muscle groups, and to the fact that movements are never performed in exactly the same way twice. This flexibility problem is demonstrated in the following example (borrowed from Raibert 1977) (Fig. 11.2).

Figure 11.2 clearly shows that an individual retains the same unique style of writing regardless of the employed muscle set (writing with the right hand, writing with the wrist immobilized, writing with the left hand, or even writing with the pen gripped between the teeth or taped to the foot). This example indicates that we are able to perform novel movements immediately. It has also been demonstrated that intelligible speech can be produced when the articulators responsible for the act are obstructed, requiring the use of different vocal tract configurations to achieve the desired phonation.

These examples emphasize complexity and plasticity, and are difficult to understand in terms of simple (muscle-specific) control models. The basic question is, how does the brain 'know' how to control these novel movements?

The storage problem

Both open-loop and closed-loop notions accept implicitly the idea of a separate trace or motor programme for each movement: a one-to-one mapping between stored states and performed movements. For example, in Adams's closed-loop theory it is clearly proposed that the reference (the perceptual trace) develops through a learning process separately for each

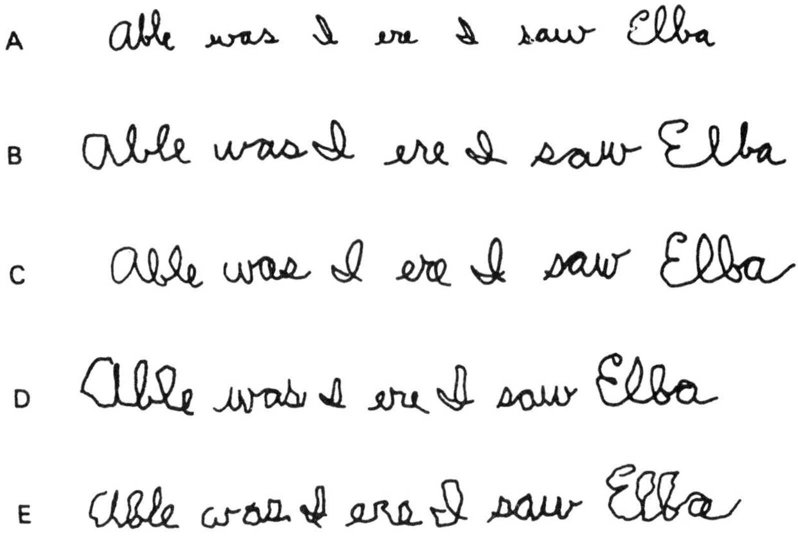

A   *able was I ere I saw Elba*

B   *Able was I ere I saw Elba*

C   *Able was I ere I saw Elba*

D   *Able was I ere I saw Elba*

E   *Able was I ere I saw Elba*

Fig. 11.2. shows 5 different ways of writing the same sentence. In A writing is with the right (dominant) hand, in B writing is with the right arm, with wrist immobilized, in C writing is with the left hand, in D the pen was gripped between the teeth, and in E the pen was taped to the foot. The figure clearly shows the muscle independency of motor control (from Raibert 1977 in Schmidt 1988).

movement. However, if there exists a separate model or reference in memory for every movement, our central nervous system should possess an almost inexhaustible storage capacity. For the speech production area, it was estimated by MacNeilage and MacNeilage (1973) that for the English language 100 000 phonemes were required, and thus the same number of stored states. When we add this to the countless ways in which human beings move their musculature, the individual must have an inexhaustible supply of either motor programmes or feedback states. Although there is no evidence that this is not the case, it is scientifically more parsimonious to suggest mechanisms that do not need this amount of storage room.

Motor learning: the acquisition of action schemata

The above-mentioned theories, in fact, represent the classical view on motor control. The nervous system is viewed as a gigantic warehouse of representations (perceptual traces, motor programmes) of every movement the individual can possibly perform. The selection of movements is accomplished by selecting from the warehouse those movement-representations that should be activated to fit one's immediate needs.

The problem with this view is obvious, and has already been mentioned. Since we are capable of performing an almost infinite number of movements it is extremely unlikely that our nervous system stores the representations of each specific movement. Therefore we are forced to accept a *constructional view* on motor control. Movement-representations are not available in ready-made form, but have to be constructed according to stored rules. Hence, it is not the final 'products' which are stored, but the rules for constructing them.

The constructional view: action schemata

The schema theory was presented by Schmidt (1975) to provide an answer to the above-mentioned problems. Schmidt rejected the idea of a one-to-one mapping between programmes and movements and suggested the existence of generalized motor programmes and schemata.

The schema idea, originally stated with respect to perception, is that in order to perceive a set of visual stimuli and to classify these stimuli correctly in a certain category we need not have previously perceived the particular set of stimuli in question. The following example (borrowed from Schmidt 1975) can explain this: when you see a dog, how do you know this animal is a dog even if you did not see this particular dog before? (Think of the analogy with movement flexibility: how can you perform a movement you never made before?) A one-to-one mapping approach would accept the storage of a visual image of each dog you ever saw. However, this cannot explain the correct identification of a totally new dog. The idea is that you do not store 'dogs' in memory, but prototypical abstract knowledge about dogs. The 'broadness' of this knowledge depends on how many different types of dogs you have seen in your life. This prototypical knowledge is termed the *schema*.

Schema-formation

How does a schema develop? Basically, when the individual makes a movement four things are stored in memory:

— *The initial conditions*: information about the muscular system and the environment.
— *The response specifications*: speed, accuracy, force, direction.
— *The sensory consequences*: the response-produced sensory information, that is, the actual feedback from eyes, ears, and proprioceptors.
— *Response outcome*: information about the success of the response in relation to the outcome originally intended.

These four sources of information are stored after the movement is produced. When a number of such movements has been made an abstract relationship between the four sources develops. The strength of the relationship increases with each successive movement of the same response class, and is strongy correlated with the accuracy of the feedback information. This abstract relationship is the *schema.*

The motor programme redefined

To solve the storage problem Schmidt (1975, 1976) introduced the concept of a *generalized motor programme* regulating a class or category of movements. For example, there are no x motor programmes for the x ways of throwing a ball, but a single programme for this category of movements. The generalized motor programme is considered as an abstract memory structure representing a raw, prototypical programme. By manipulating various parameters (or response specifications) the same programme can be employed for several movement outcomes. For example, by changing the parameter *force* the same 'throwing programme' can be used for throwing an object over various distances. By means of the *schema rules* these parameters are selected.

Much is unknown about the content of such a programme. According to some authors it contains information concerning the temporal structure of the action (Van Galen and Teulings 1983; Van Galen and Wing 1984) or force–time relationshps (Schmidt 1980), or 'topological' information (Bernstein 1967).

Keele (1981) presented a version of the motor programme in which the programme controls the proper sequence of the action to be generated. In the present chapter it is also argued that the main function of a motor programme is to regulate the order of the action elements. For example, consider the writing of the letter 'L'. The normal sequence is from top to bottom and then from left to right. However, it can be written large or small, with the left or the right hand, etc. Hence the actual execution of the movement is extremely flexible. It seems logical to argue that the employed muscles are not specified in the programme, as they are too variable, and depend largely on the actual current requirements. Hence, the order is programmed, but not the specific muscles. Which muscles are chosen forms a 'lower order' control problem, and depends on environmental conditions.

Rehabilitation therapy as the (re-)acquisition of action schemata

Schmidt (1975, 1976) argued that the learning of motor skills could be understood in terms of the acquisition of schemata or rules. This idea was a fundamental break in the tradition whereby motor learning was considered to be the establishment of specific perceptual traces or muscle-specific motor programmes which defined only a particular movement. The schema theory implied that motor programmes were generalized, and that complex rules had to be formed to run these programmes.

This theory has clear implications for rehabilitation therapy. The development of a schema is positively influenced by the following factors:

- Variability of practice
- The consistent use of feedback
- A close relationship between the therapy and the activities of daily living
- The emphasis on active movements instead of passive guidance

Variability of practice

If during motor learning we are acquiring action schemata, this implies that learning by means of repetition of separate movements will be useless. Indeed, as in the case of 'dog recognition', a rich (movement) experience is necessary to develop a schema. In other words, if therapy is the acquisition of schemata or prototypical knowledge about the skill under training, then it is predicted that the 'quality' of the acquired schema depends largely on the variability of practice. Patients receiving variability of practice should perform novel motor tasks (within the same response class) better than patients who were exercised under a constant practice regime (repetition of the same correct movement). Experimental evidence for this prediction has been found, particularly with children (Shapiro and Schmidt 1982). Perhaps this can be explained from the fact that in most of the experiments the tasks were very simple. Hence, adults had already established the schemata for performing these simple experimental tasks. Therefore no real learning (schema-formation), was required. For the children the situation was different. Since they did not possess a large set of already developed schemata, for them the situation possessed a clear learning component. However, therapy with patients suffering from motor disorders also contains a large learning component—patients have to acquire novel motor skills—and in this context the variability of practice seems to be still valid.

Rule 1: Therapy, in so far as it concerns motor learning, should be structured in such a way that practice takes place in a variable context.

The consistent use of feedback

Normally our movements are accompanied by a continuous 'stream' of afferent information. If the movement does not feel right, we try to adapt and correct the movement. The archer can see if the arrow is missing the target, and can compensate in the next response. Even before we see the actual result of the movement we have an idea concerning the quality of it.

People suffering from the consequences of damage to the central nervous system often do not have these normal sources of sensory feedback any longer. They are not aware what they do wrong to cause an imperfect response, because their feedback loops are disturbed. In this case it is necessary for the therapist to provide relevant information. Without *knowledge of results* (KR) improvement cannot occur. Without knowledge of results it is very difficult to develop an action schema, since feedback (response outcome) is one of the four essential sources of information stored after a response. Knowledge of results about the outcome of an action is one of the most potent variables in learning. The knowledge of results provides information to the performer, who evaluates this in relation to the desired goal. Designers of learning situations, as therapists are, should do everything possible to ensure that such information is available to patients (Mulder 1985; Mulder and Hulstijn, 1985, 1988).

The following practical implications can be derived from the literature on feedback and learning. First, feedback is essential for improving performance, and the more the better (see Schmidt *et al.* 1990 for a critical analysis of KR). But the feedback trials should be interspersed with no-feedback trials, so that the subjects are forced to learn to perform the task without the guidance provided by the feedback. Presenting information on every other trial or every third trial might be an effective method. Dependency on feedback should be avoided. Second, knowledge of results should be provided as soon after completion of the response as possible. This will maximize the learner's ability to associate the estimated response outcome information with the actual results of the performed movement. Third, the interval between the presentation of the feedback and the start of a new attempt should be kept relatively free of other movements that could be confused with the target movement(s). Fourth, since the learner needs time to 'construct' a new response, he/she should not be interrupted during the post-KR interval. Presumably, the more complex the task, the more critical the time needed for information processing. Learning appears to suffer from too short or filled post-KR intervals (see above).

Feedback: information or motivation?

Often the role of feedback has been described in terms of motivation. In this view the knowledge of results functions as an external reward, reinforcing the correct response. However, numerous lines of evidence suggest that humans do not use the feedback as a reinforcer or a motivational cue, but as a source of information about what to do next (Adams 1971). This information-processing orientation of feedback has important practical implications. Knowing that feedback is primarily informational will tend to bias therapists away from post-response statements such as 'nice job' (reward) to statements containing more information concerning the desired outcome.

Rule 2: Therapy should be structured in such a way that knowledge of results is always available for the patient, especially at the beginning of the learning process.

Verbal instructions and demonstrations

The most popular methods for conveying information about the goal and appropriate action sequences are verbal instructions and demonstrations. To instil in the learner the nature and the goal of the act therapists often resort to demonstrations. This is either accomplished live by the therapist or a filmed demonstration may be given, with or without augmented instructions. There is evidence that modelling techniques are important for the acquisition of motor skills. For example, Landers (1975) performed a study employing the Bachman ladder. Three groups had to climb the free-standing ladder as high as possible. All the groups received verbal instructions, but the groups differed in terms of when an additional live modelling demonstration was given. One group was given the demonstration before any practice began, the second group was given the demonstration midway through the practice sequence, and the third group was given the demonstration both before and midway through practice. The results showed that the two groups who received modelling before the start of practice performed more effectively than the group who started with only the instruction. In another study Landers and Landers (1973) showed that, while for low-skilled subjects the use of a peer model was more effective than the use of a teacher model, the reverse was true for high-skilled subjects.

Several authors indicated the relevance of observational learning for the motor skills area (Carroll and Bandura 1982, 1985; Whiting *et al.* 1987). It is therefore surprising to discover that in therapy this learning procedure (using video tapes or live models) is hardly employed, since the human being is particularly well 'equipped' to transform observations immediately into the correct actions. Meltzoff and Moore (1977) described how new-borns are already able to imitate facial expressions, that is, are able to translate visual information immediately into motor patterns. In very much the same way patients who have reached a certain level of functioning can be employed as models for patients who had not reached this level. The latter patients can be instructed to imitate the 'more highly skilled' subjects.

Rule 3: Therapy should make more use of observational learning procedures.

A close relationship between the therapy and the activities of daily living

Recall that it was argued that separate movements play no role in the learning process. No muscle-specific combinations are learned, but goal-directed actions. These actions are represented in memory by means of action schemata. However, the usefulness of these action schemata depends largely on the structure of the therapy. A therapy focused on the level of muscles and movements, that is, aimed at restoring distorted elements instead of distorted actions, will result in the development of a very 'narrow' schema. Such a 'narrow' schema is of almost no use in daily life. To improve the generalization-value of the acquired schema a patient should be exercised in a situation resembling as closely as possible the daily world. If the gap between the therapeutic situation and the daily-life situation is large, the schema acquired during therapy will be of no use for the activities of daily life. The number of identical elements across the two situations is too limited, so that almost no transfer takes place from one to the other learning situation. Hence, a therapy separated from daily-life situations creates an artificial learning situation with minimal long-term effects.

Rule 4: Therapy should be structured in such a way that a maximum overlap is realized between the therapy situation and the daily-life situation ('law of identical elements')

Active movements vs *passive guidance*

A technique frequently used in therapy involves guidance, whereby the learner is in some way guided through the task. Although such a procedure may have positive effects on the mechanical condition of the muscular system, it has hardly any learning effect (Newell 1981; Levitt 1982). A major conceptual problem with guidance in a learning context is that it eliminates the learner's need to select the appropriate response.

Rule 5: Passive movement does not result in learning.

Stages in learning

Three stages can be distinguished in the learning process (Fitts 1964). The first stage is termed the *verbal motor stage* or the *cognitive stage.* During this first phase the patient has to understand the meaning and the goal of the therapy. Considerable cognitive activity is required—good strategies have to be retained whereas inappropriate ones have to be discarded. During this phase the performance of the patient is usually very inconsistent, because he or she tries many different ways to reach the goal. It is extremely important that in this first phase the therapist provides the patient with sufficient sources of feedback. During the first phase of the therapy process a global idea concerning the correct action has to be developed, a cognitive representation that can function as an internal model or reference for action. The feedback of the action is compared against the internal model. If at this stage such information is not available or is insufficient or inconsistent the development of such a crude first reference is impossible. It is the therapist's responsibility to deliver this information.

Verbal activity from the side of the learner plays an important role in this first phase. The learner uses self-instruction as a method to guide his attempts.

The second phase in the acquisition process is termed the *motor stage* or *association phase*. This phase starts when the individual has acquired an effective way of performing. The performance is more consistent, and the attentional load of the task has been reduced. Practice should take place in a daily-life setting, so as to strengthen the schema further.

The third stage is termed the *autonomous phase*. Now, the skill has become more or less automatic. Sometimes it takes hundreds or thousands of repetitions to reach this final phase.

Recent developments in motor control theories

The notions so far discussed are all *cognitive*, that is to say, they all accept the existence of a complex set of internal (mental) processes. Some psychologists have criticized this approach, and defend a more biomechanical notion based on the work of the Russian scientist Bernstein (see Kelso 1982, part V). Bernstein discussed the study of movement in terms of the problems of co-ordinating and controlling a complex system of biokinematic links. He understood that the focus of analysis could not simply be the muscular forces provided by the organism, but must include inertia or reactive forces. Bernstein's work was focused on the *degrees of freedom* problem. This problem constitutes a very difficult and fundamental puzzle for students of movement. The problem is also of relevance for rehabilitation therapy.

As we have seen, Schmidt (1975) solved the degrees of freedom problem by introducing the schema as a cognitive concept. The Bernsteinian approach takes another route. Consider the control of an individual arm. The arm consists of shoulder, elbow, radio-ulnar, and wrist joints. Now consider we want to control this arm, what sort of problems do we meet (the example is borrowed from Turvey *et al.* 1982, pp. 241–2)? The shoulder joint can move on three axes, that is to say when the arm is fully extended it can still vary its position to the right and left and upward and downward, and it can rotate about its length. Hence, the shoulder joint has three degrees of freedom. The elbow has only one degree of freedom, whereas the wrist joint has two degrees of freedom. Considering that the units of control are the joints, then the central executive has a problem to solve with 7 degrees of freedom.

Now consider the muscles as the units of control. In that case the problem is much more complicated, since there are 10 muscles working around the shoulder joint, 6 muscles working at the elbow, 4 muscles are responsible for the working of the radio-ulnar joint, and finally 6 muscles move the wrist. Here we have a problem with 26 degrees of freedom. The control problem is of bewildering complexity for theories accepting the individual motor units as the elements of control. Hence, the key problem for the central nervous system is how to reduce the degrees of freedom problem, or in other words how to reduce the control problem. An interesting hypothesis is that nature solves this puzzle for us by keeping the degrees of freedom individually controlled at a minimum by using 'functional units' defined over the motor system that automatically adjust to each other and to changes in the field of external forces.

These functional units (also termed co-ordinative structures) develop during a learning process. Turvey *et al.* described the difference between a novice in shooting and a skilled marksman. What makes these two persons different? When observing the novice it can be seen that the arm is not stable, there is a tremor, and the muscles are not 'linked' to each other. The skilled marksman, on the other hand, is able to stabilize the body. Deviations in one part of the muscle–joint complex (for example, the wrist) are immediately compensated by a movement in the shoulder. Hence, the muscle–joint complex functions as a unit. What previously was a system with many degrees of freedom (the relatively independent function of the separate muscle–joint combinations in the novice) now becomes a system of fewer degrees of freedom. Here we have a fundamental principle which states that the number of degrees of freedom of the system controlling action is much less than the number of mechanical degrees of freedom of the controlled system (Turvey 1977). Learning can be characterized as a process directed at reducing the degrees of freedom, and at the development of co-ordinative structures.

Co-ordinative structures have their origins in the relative autonomous subsystems of the spinal cord. The role of higher levels of the nervous system is to modulate interactions within and among neural mechanisms at the spinal level. It is important to note that this system of segmental interactions can be 'prejudiced' towards executive intentions. The process of biasing is termed tuning. Tuning can, for example, take place by means of visual input. This optical input (recall Lee's experiments described earlier in this text) tunes or prepares the spinal control systems. Optical information can affect muscle reflexes in human subjects.

Take, for example, the following experiment, in which subjects were asked to fall forward, hands first, on to a platform. The platform could be tilted at various angles away from the body. The EMG acivity in the m. triceps was monitored during the self-initiated fall toward the platform. When subjects were able to see the platform, the time of the onset of the EMG activity varied, so that it always began a constant amount of time before impact, regardless how far away the platform was. However, if the subjects were blindfolded, and had no way of knowing when impact would occur, the muscle response-time was stereotyped, starting always at the beginning of the fall (Dietz and Noth 1978).

Not only perceptual systems can tune the muscle system, but also the muscle systems can tune each other. As you turn your head to one side, there is a bias toward extending the arm on the side of the body to which your head is turned and a bias toward flexing the arm on the opposite side. Hence, as one part of the body changes with reference to another part, a tuning of the spinal organization takes place.

Gelfand *et al.* (1971) argue that the control of movement is in many aspects the reorganization or tuning of the system of segmental interactions, and that this attunement precedes the transmission of activating instructions to co-ordinative structures. A motion like stepping or raising the arm is anticipated through supraspinal tuning of the segmental mechanisms.

The relationship between cognitive theories and the concept of co-ordinative structures

How do the theoretical notions as described in the last section relate to the cognitive notions described earlier in the text? It is a difficult question to answer, since the theories start from different premises. As was mentioned, the cognitive approach accepts a hierarchy of internal processes functioning in the time-interval between stimulus and response, whereas the co-ordinative structure does not accept such an information-processing approach. There is no experimental evidence which unambiguously supports one notion and rejects the other. One could even wonder if such a crucial experiment is possible.

A possible answer to the above-mentioned question could be that the type of control employed by the system ('direct' control *vs* cognitive processing) is dependent on the type of task. For example regulating balance while standing and playing a saxophone could be very well explained by means of co-ordinative structures (optical information tunes the segmental system of the cord). But can we also explain how it is possible to play 'Rhapsody in blue' without notes and still denying any mental concept (for example, stored information)? It can be argued that in tasks with a heavy learning component, such as playing a musical instrument, the cognitive approach cannot be missed out, whereas in tasks such as standing, walking, etc. the explanation can be given in terms of a more direct control. However, where standing balance has to be re-acquired, as after lower limb amputation, it appears that the early phases are under the control of cognitive processes (Geurts *et al.* 1991; Geurts *et al.*, in press).

Since rehabilitation therapy, for a large part, can be viewed as a learning process the cognitive approach seems to be valid. A further advantage of the cognitive approach is that operationalization in an experimental context is possible. Hence, the approach is 'testable'.

A last remark concerns the difference between the two notions. Although in several publications it is suggested that the two notions are totally opposed to each other, I think this is a useless dichotomy. In fact, the two frameworks are completing each other. Human motor behaviour is regulated by means of a hybrid control system.

Conclusion

Recent notions on motor control and learning have been discussed. However, many questions remain. As already mentioned in the introduction, no definite answers can be given. The primary purpose of the present text was to give the reader an impression of modern psychological thinking on motor control and learning. We have seen that the learning of motor control can be understood in terms of the acquisition of abstract plans or rules (or ways to link muscle–joint systems).

Visual information, feedback, variability of practice, active movements, and ecologically valid context all play a role in this acquisition process. These requirements can be seen as *instruments* in the hands of a therapist, and can be employed in the development of a modern therapy.

The confrontation between psychology and the field of rehabilitation is too young to expect definite answers, but it can open new perspectives for therapy and research.

References

Adams, J. A. (1971). A closed loop theory of motor learning. *Journal of Motor Behavior*, **3**, 111–50.

Bernstein, N. (1967). *The coordination and regulation of movement.* Pergamon, London.

Bles, W. and Brandt, Th. (1986). *Disorders of posture and gait.* Elsevier, Amsterdam.

Brandt, Th., Wenzel, D., and Dichgans, J. (1976). Die Entwicklung der visuellen Stabilisation des aufrechten Standes beim Kind: ein Reifezeichen in der Kinder neurologie. *Archiv. für Psychiatrie und Nervenkrankheiten*, **223**, 1–13.

Butterworth, G. and Hicks, L. (1977). Visual proprioception and postural stability in infancy: a developmental study. *Perception*, **6**, 255–62.

Carroll, W. R. and Bandura, A. (1982). The role of visual monitoring in observational learning of action patterns: making the unobservable observable. *Journal of Motor Behavior*, **14**, 153–67.

Carroll, W. R. and Bandura, A. (1985). Role of timing of visual monitoring and motor rehearsal in observational learning of action patterns. *Journal of Motor Behavior*, **17**, 269–83.

Dichgans, J., Diener, H. C., and Brandt, Th. (1974). Optokinetic–graviceptive interaction in different head positions. *Acta Oto-Laryngologica*, **78**, 391–8.

Dietz, V. and Noth, J. (1978). Pre-innervation and stretch responses of triceps brachii in man falling with and without visual control. *Brain Research*, **142**, 576–9.

Fitts, P. M. (1964). Perceptual-motor skills learning. In *Categories of human learning* (ed. A. W. Melton), pp. 243–85. Academic Press, New York.

Gelfand, I. M., Gurfinkel, V. S., Tsetlin, M. L., and Shik, M. L. (1971). In *Models of the structural functional organization of certain biological systems* (ed. I. M. Gelfand, V. S. Gurfinkel, S. V. Fomin, and M. L. Tsetlin), pp. 329–45. MIT Press, Cambridge, Massachusetts.

Geurts, A. C. H., Mulder, Th., Nienhuis, B., and Ryken, R. (1991). From the analysis of movement to the analysis of skills: bridging the gap between the laboratory and the clinic. *Journal of Rehabilitation Sciences*, **4**, 9–13.

Geurts, A. C. H., Mulder, Th., Nienhuis, B., and Ryken, R. Dual task assessment of reorganisation of postural control in persons with lower limb amputation. *Archives of Physical Medicine and Rehabilitation* (in press.)

Gibson, J. J. (1979). *The ecological approach to visual perception.* Houghton Mifflin, Boston.

Hocherman, S. and Dickstein, R. (1984). Platform training and postural stability in hemiplegics. *Archives of Physical Medicine and Rehabilitation*, **65**, 588–92.

Hulstijn, W. and Mulder, Th. (1985). Stoornisen in de fijne motoriek: en poging tot diagnostiek. In *Studies over schrijfmotoriek* (ed. A. J. W. M. Thomassen, G. P. Van Galen, and L. F. De Klerk), pp. 229–43.

Hulstijn, W. and Mulder, Th. (1986). Motor dysfunctions in children: toward a process oriented diagnosis. In *Themes in motor development* (ed. H. T. A. Whiting and M. G. Wade), pp. 109–26.

Keele, S. W. (1968). Movement control in skilled motor performance. *Psychological Bulletin*, **70**, 387–403.

Keele, S. W. (1981). Behavioral analysis of movement. In *Handbook of physiology*, Section 1, *The nervous system*. Vol. 2, part 2: *Motor control* (ed. V. B. Brooks), pp. 1391–1414. American Physiological Society, Bethesda, Maryland.

Kelso, J. A. S. (1982). *Human motor behavior: an introduction.* Erlbaum, Hillsdale.

Landers, D. M. (1975). Observational learning of a motor skill: temporal spacing of demonstrations and audience present. *Journal of Motor Behavior*, **5**, 281–7.

Landers, D. M. and Landers, D. M. (1973). Teacher versus peer models: effect of model's presence and performance level on motor behavior. *Journal of Motor Behavior*, **5**, 129–39.

Lee, D. N. (1980). Visuo-motor coordination in space time. In *Tutorials in motor behavior* (ed. G. E. Stelmach and J. Requin), pp. 281–97. North-Holland, Amsterdam.

Lee, D. N. and Aronson, E. (1974). Visual proprioceptive control of stance in human infants. *Perception and Psychophysics*, **15**, 527–32.

Lee, D. N. and Reddish, P. E. (1981). Plummeting gannets: a paradigm for ecological optics. *Nature*, **5830**, 293–4.

Lee, D. N., Lishman, J. R., and Thomson, J. A. (1982). Regulation of gait in long-jumpers. *Journal of Experimental Psychology: Human perception and performance*, **8**, 448–59.

Levitt, S. (1982). *Treatment of cerebral palsy and motor delay.* Blackwell, Oxford.

Lincoln, N. B., Whiting, S. E., Cockburn, J., and Bhavnani, G. (1985). An evaluation of perceptual training. *International Journal of Rehabilitation Medicine*, **7**, 99–101.

MacNeilage, P. F. and MacNeilage, L. A. (1973). Central processes controlling speech production during sleep and waking. In *The psychophysiology of thinking* (ed. F. J. McGuigan), pp. 417–48. Academic Press, New York.

Meltzoff, A. N. and Moore, M. K. (1977). Imitation of facial and manual gestures by human neonates. *Science*, **118**, 75–88.

Mulder, Th. (1985). *The learning of motor control following brain damage: experimental and clinical studies.* Swets & Zeitlinger, Lisse.

Mulder, Th. and Hulstijn, W. (1984). Sensory feedback therapy and theoretical knowledge of motor control and learning. *American Journal of Physical Medicine*, **63**, 226–44.

Mulder, Th. and Hulstijn, W. (1985). Sensory feedback therapy and the learning of a novel motor task. *Journal of Motor Behavior*, **17**, 110–28.

Mulder, Th. and Hulstijn, W. (1988). From movement to action: the learning of motor control following brain damage. In *Complex movement behaviour: 'the' motor-action controversy* (ed. O. G. Meijer and K. Roth), pp. 247–61. North-Holland, Amsterdam.

Mulder, Th., Hulstijn, W., and van de Bunte, A. (1986). Motorische stoornissen bij kinderen: de ontwikkeling van een diagnostische taak. *Nederlands Tijdschrift voor de Psychologie*, **41**, 48–55.

Nashner, L. M. and Berthoz, A. (1978). Visual contribution to rapid motor responses during postural control. *Brain Research*, **150**, 403–7.

Newell, K. M. (1981). Skill learning. In *Human skills* (ed. D. Holding), pp. 203–26. Wiley, London.

Pew, R. W. (1966). Acquisition of hierarchical control over temporal organization of a skill. *Journal of Experimental Psychology*, **71**, 764–71.

Raibert, M. H. (1977). *Motor control and learning by the state–space model.* Technical Report, Artificial Intelligence Laboratory, MIT (AI-TR-439).

Schmidt, R. A. (1975). A schema theory of discrete motor learning. *Psychological Review*, **82**, 225–61.

Schmidt, R. A. (1976). The schema as a solution to some persistent problems in motor learning theory. In *Motor control: issues and trends* (ed. G. E. Stelmach), pp. 43–65. Academic Press, New York.

Schmidt, R. A. (1980). On the theoretical status of time in motor-program representations. In *Tutorials in motor behavior* (ed. G. E. Stelmach and J. Requin), pp. 145–67. North-Holland, Amsterdam.

Schmidt, R. A. (1988). *Motor control and learning: a behavioral emphasis.* Human Kinetics, Champaign.

Schmidt, R. A., Lange, C., and Young, D. E. (1990). Optimizing summary knowledge of results for skill learning. *Human Movement Science*, **9**, 325–48.

Shapiro, D. C. and Schmidt, R. A. (1982). The schema theory: recent evidence and developmental implications. In *The development of motor control and coordination* (ed. J. A. S. Kelso and J. E. Clark), pp. 113–51. Wiley, New York.

Thoden, E., Dichgans, J., and Savadis, Th. (1977). Direction specific optokinetic modulation of monosynaptic hindlimb reflexes in cats. *Experimental Brain Research*, **30**, 13–24.

Turvey, M. T. (1977). Preliminaries to a theory of action with reference to vision. In *Perceiving, acting and knowing: toward an ecological psychology* (ed. R. Shaw and J. Bransford), pp. 211–65. Erlbaum, Hillsdale.

Turvey, M. T., Fitc, H. L., and Tulle, B. (1982). The Bernstein perspective: the problem of degrees of freedom and context-conditioned variability. In *Human motor behavior: an introduction* (ed. J. A. S. Kelso), pp. 239–52. Erlbaum, Hillsdale.

van Galen, G. P. and Teulings, H. L. (1983). The independent monitoring of form and scale factors in handwriting. *Acta psychologia*, **54**, 9–22.

van Galen, G. P. and Wing, A. M. (1984). The sequencing of movements. In *The psychology of human movement* (ed. M. M. Smyth and A. M. Wing), pp. 153–83. Academic Press, New York.

van Ravensberg, C. D., Tyldesley, D. A., Rozendal, R. H., and Whiting, H. T. A. (1984). Visual perception in hemiplegic patients. *Archives of Physical Medicine and Rehabilitation*, **65**, 304–9.

Wadman, W. J., Denier van der Gon, J. J., Geuze, R. H., and Mol, C. R. (1979). Control of fast goal-directed arm movements. *Journal of Human Movement Studies*, **5**, 3–17.

Whiting, H. T. A., Bijlard, M. J., and den Brinker, B. (1987). The effect of the availability of a dynamic model on the acquisition of a complex cyclical action. *Quarterly Journal of Experimental Psychology*, **39A**, 153–67

Woollacott, M. H. (1986). Postural control and development. In *Themes in motor development* (ed. H. T. A. Whiting and M. G. Wade), pp. 3–21. Nijhoff, The Hague.

Young, L. R., Oman, C. M., and Dichgans, J. (1975). Influence of head orientation on visually induced pitch and roll sensation. *Aviation, Space and Environmental Medicine*, **46**, 264–8.

12

Rehabilitation

L. S. Illis

Rehabilitation implies the use of medical, social, educational, and vocational measures for restoring the individual to the highest level of physical, mental, and social ability in the shortest possible time. In most cases of spinal cord dysfunction the nature of the lesion or disease is such that rehabilitation must involve a continuing programme, although the degree of involvement may vary from time to time.

Although the future, as regards patients with spinal injury, must lie in the fields of regrowth and connection of nerve fibres and in the development of genetic engineering techniques to encourage growth connection, there is real evidence for improved function using new approaches to intervention and treatment. However, any improvement produced by various therapies will give only limited benefit if physical therapy measures are not utilized as well. The highest level of functional ability must be maintained: for example, regrowth of nerve fibres will not suffice to restore function if the patient cannot sustain weight-bearing or joint-movement, or contractures have occurred.

All rehabilitation measures must rely upon accurate assessment. This is essential in order to plan rehabilitation programmes and to delineate goals, and also as a means of monitoring progress and validating therapy. Clinical and physiological assessment has been dealt with in Volume I (*Spinal cord dysfunction: assessment*). There are many clinical assessment schedules, but, unfortunately, no general accepted disability assessment, and most re-habilitation units use a locally adapted schedule. Although this is useful for the individual unit, it becomes impossible to compare the outcome of therapy from unit to unit.

The untreated patient

Completely untreated patients are rare. However, it is worth bearing in mind that an untreated tetraplegic who is unable to cough effectively will drown in his own secretions within the first few days after injury, or may develop ileus and dilatation of the stomach, and is likely to die of inhalation of vomit. Paraplegics will almost certain develop severe pressure sores with secondary infection and urinary tract infection. Osteomyelitis and septicaemia will ensue, and the few patients who survive this will die of urinary tract complications on a background of increasing contractures and spasticity.

Early intervention and treatment

The stage of mobilization will depend upon the presence or otherwise of fracture or fracture dislocation in spinal-injured patients. Where there is no such disturbance the aim is to mobilize the patient as early as possible. Where bed-rest is essential, nursing on a special turning bed should avoid the occurrence of pressure areas. Posturing and positioning is carried out in such a way as to keep muscles, joints, and limbs in a neutral position in order to avoid contractures, with frequent corrections of the patient's position. It is a truism that rehabilitation starts as soon as the injury or lesion occurs, and the importance of this is best seen in the care of joints and muscles, since contractures are likely to become pronounced within the first few weeks if treatment is delayed.

Passive and active movement is not only necessary from the points of view of preventing pressure areas and improving cardio-vascular function, but also in the prevention of para-articular ossification.

Eventually the paralysed limbs will begin to demineralize, and as a result paralysed patients are prone to fracture of legs, sometimes from relatively minor trauma. The progress of demineralization can be prevented to some extent by regular weight-bearing.

Where a high spinal cord lesion has occurred blood-pressure control may be impaired or abolished, and it is necessary to mobilize the patient very slowly into the sitting position, with careful monitoring of blood-pressure. Sometimes it is necessary to use limb cuffs.

The more specific aspects of rehabilitation should be a joint effort by the therapist and the patient. Important aspects such as spasticity, the management of cardio-vascular abnormalities, bladder management, the treatment of pain, and the treatment of infertility are dealt with in detail earlier in this volume, and these accounts will not be reiterated here.

The treatment of skin care is a good example of the importance of the involvement of both patient and therapist. The patient must be fully aware of the fact that lack of sensation is likely to produce pressure sores. The patient must be taught to alter posture and to lift the body for short periods and at regular intervals. Daily inspection of skin over pressure areas is an important part of prophylaxis, and this must be explained to the patient.

Family and social care

The degree of family and social care which can be provided and which is necessary depends partly on the disability caused by the lesion, but also on factors which include financial status, the presence or absence of family members, and the presence of available social security. The failure of family support and social security is probably the greatest reason for institutional care. Domiciliary services should be instigated as early as possible, since architectural adaptation in terms of handrails, alteration of bath and lavatory accommodation, etc., may be necessary.

Counselling

Counselling should include practical information both to the patient and to the family. It involves continuous advice and guidance and, where necessary, support. Obviously time must be set aside for communication between the doctor in charge of the case, the patient, and the family; but the need for continual counselling must be recognized by all members of the therapeutic team. Counselling is at all levels, including, for example, the need for skin care, the management of bladder disability, advice about social security, etc.

Group discussions between disabled patients are often useful, and in some instances groups of relatives or families may give active support to each other as well as to patients. Many disability groups have support associations. Holebrook (1982) has proposed a model for the adjustment of disability similar to models which have been put forward for bereavement. Holebrook identifies four stages describing the reaction of families to patients with stroke illness. In the first stage, 'crisis', there are the reactions of shock, confusion, and anxiety. In the second stage, the 'treatment stage', there is often a high expectation of recovery, a denial of permanent disability, grieving, and fears for the future, including the future as regards mobility, life-style, the ability to cope, and employment. In the third stage, 'realization of disability', reactions include anger, rejection, despair, frustration, and depression. The final stage is that of adjustment. If the doctor in charge of the patient and the therapeutic team recognize these stages and the reactions that occur, then counselling of the patient and the family is likely to be more logical and more successful.

Physiotherapy

The techniques of physiotherapy are frequently dismissed by doctors as being relatively unremarkable, and simply used 'as appropriate'. For example, putting joints through a range of passive movements. However, physiotherapy techniques include not only the prevention of complications in the limbs which are not functioning or poorly functioning, or training normal muscles to compensate for loss of function, but also are involved in attempts to overcome the disability in paralysed limbs. These newer techniques are often called 'facilitation therapy' or 'inhibition therapy', and are as much a part of modern physiotherapy as passive movements, massage, and active exercises. Many of the facilitation and inhibition techniques were based, or were intended to be based, upon neurophysiological studies; and they were all developed as treatment for patients with cerebral problems rather than for those with spinal dysfunction.

Patients with spinal dysfunction have no particular school devoted to them, such as those named and briefly described below. However, many of the techniques which suppress spasticity, alter abnormal reflex activity, and relieve spasm and pain are clearly applicable to patients with spinal dysfunction. Although the followers of particular schools emphasize the differences between them, the general principles are actually much the same. The major facilitation techniques were described by Fay (1948), Kabat (1952), Rood (1954), Knott (1967), Brunnstrom (1970), and Bobath (1978). The Bobath method, and variations of it, are based on the premise that movement is continuously modulated by afferent information. Neurological lesions alter the control exerted by afferent systems and unmask abnormal reflex activity. Stimulation of afferent systems (adjustment of posture, skin-stimulation, and joint-movement) will suppress spasticity and pathological reflexes. The patient is then taught simple repetitive exercises which gradually build up to a return to controlled movement.

In the Brunnstrom approach abnormal reflex patterns are broken down using facilitation techniques or sensory stimulation, such as the stretching and tapping of muscles. Adherents deny any similarity to the Bobath method, although both schools claim their techniques are based on the same neurophysiological principles. The similarities become closer, as each school (other than purists) uses similar aids.

The proprioceptive neuro-muscular facilitation school of Kabat and Knott is again based on the precept that motor behaviour is continuously modulated by sensory information, and not many people would argue with that. Kabat designed patterns of movement intended to re-establish normal agonist–antagonist muscle action. Knott went a little further: the physiotherapist assists the patient's initial attempts at movement, so theoretically producing an afferent barrage from muscle spindles and Golgi tendon organs, i.e. 'proprioceptive neuromuscular facilitation'. As power and control improve, further training includes the application of resistance.

In the Rood method, widespread sensory stimulation is used.

These techniques, and variations of them, are widely used both by idealist adherents of a particular technique, and, more commonly, by therapists using a combination of various facilitation techniques adapted to the individual patient and the specific neurological disability. The summaries given above leave out the details of the rational basis for the various techniques. All the techniques were developed for the treatment of stroke patients, but are appropriate for spinal dysfunction. Controlled trials which evaluate these different techniques or compare the facilitation techniques to a more traditional approach are virtually non-existent. This, however, should not detract from the fact that the techniques may actually produce a certain degree of restoration of function.

The Peto Institute in Budapest has developed an approach to neurological disability which is called 'conductive education', and is said to be based on the concept of plasticity of the nervous system; that is, of the re-establishing of new patterns of connection or the opening up of paths which are not normally used. The neuro-anatomy and the neurophysiology is well established in experimental work (see Vol. I, *Spinal cord dysfunction: assessment*, 1988). There are many anecdotal accounts of the effectiveness of this kind of treatment, but there are no properly structured trials. Again, this approach was developed for patients with cerebral dysfunction.

Stimulation techniques

This is a large and gradually increasing field which started with the use of functional electrical stimulation by Liberson *et al.* (1961). This complex and wide field of therapy will be dealt with in a separate volume, since it includes stimulation techniques ranging from methods of improving blood-supply to the treatment of infertility.

Occupational therapy

There is usually some degree of ignorance as to the true role of occupational therapists in the management and treatment of patients with neurological disability. The best way of summarizing the occupational therapist's role is to say that the therapist is involved in assessing not so much the functional disability as the patient's capability after a lesion has occurred. This includes the assessment of disability and handicap and the training of the patient in various techniques, including collaborating with physiotherapists and doctors. The occupational therapist is involved in the application of aids and various tools for living and the training of patients to use them, and the education of the patient's family in the use of such techniques. The aim of occupational therapy, as with physiotherapy, is to enable the patient to return home and to live as independently as possible; and, indeed, this is the aim of all therapies.

This short résumé of rehabilitation must be seen in conjunction with earlier chapters outlining treatment and interventional techniques. Rehabilitation cannot be separated from treatment, as though it were an isolated speciality, and should be planned from the onset of the neurological insult, and continued for as long as neurological disability continues.

References

Bobath, B. (1978). *Adult hemiplegia evaluation and treatment.* Heinemann, London.

Brunnstrom, S. (1970). *Movement therapy in hemiplegia.* Harper & Row, New York.

Fay, T. (1948). The neurological aspects of therapy in cerebral palsy. *Archives of Physical Medicine,* **29**, 327–31.

Holebrook, M. (1982). Stroke: Social and emotional outcome. *Journal of the Royal College of Physicians of London,* **16**, 100–4.

Kabat, H. (1952). Studies on neuromuscular dysfunction. The role of central facilitation in restoration of motor function in paralysis. *Archives of Physical Medicine,* **33**, 521–3.

Knott, M. (1967). Introduction to and philosophy of neuromuscular facilitation. *Physiotherapy,* **53**, 2–5.

Liberson, W. T., Halmquest, H. J., Scott, D., and Dow, M. (1961). Functional electrotherapy: stimulation of the peroneal nerve synchronized with the swing phase of the gait of hemiplegic patients. *Archives of Physical Medicine,* **42**, 101–5.

Rood, M. S. (1954). Neurophysiological reactions as a basis for physical therapy. *Physical Therapy Review,* **34**, 444.

Index